TO SUICIDE AND BACK

A Real-Life Story of

Professional, Financial, and mental crisis

BY PEYMAN PEJMAN

&

JACK C. LENNON

Prologue

In November 2019, a fifty-five-year-old Chinese man from the Hubei province, who has not been named publicly, reportedly caught a virus that no one knew much about. He died later, but again we do not know the details. In less than a month, there were twenty-seven similar cases. By sometime in January 2020, there was a widespread epidemic of what we now know to be the coronavirus, or COVID-19, in the central Chinese city of Wuhan. By March, half the world was suffering from a virus about which no one knew much, for which there was no vaccine or medicine, and which had taken all governments by surprise, all scrambling to provide the essential medical facilities and logistics.

By mid-April, governments had shut down businesses and people were being furloughed or outright fired. Tens of millions of people around the world were suffering not only from worsening financial hardships, but also from the psychological pressures of stay-at-home orders, social-distancing, and limited mobility.

That's where this book comes in—hopefully! Depending on who you are and what you are going through, this book can be relevant to two types of people.

For years, friends have been telling me to write a memoir. I always refused, saying something to the tune of "Who am I to write a memoir?" I still don't think that my life has been significant enough to deserve a memoir, but I hope that the format of this book will prove enticing enough to tell the bigger story without my having written a "me" book!

Then, as you will see in the following pages, life put me through the most challenging test I have ever been through. I planned to commit suicide. I had researched the drug, where to buy it, how much I needed, and how to inject it. But I survived. How? I suppose it was a combination of fate and the kind of inner and indestructible resolve that is synonymous with the life story of millions and millions of immigrants who uproot themselves from one culture, replant, nourish, and grow stronger roots in another country, another culture. That experience and uncompromising attitude alone builds a certain resiliency that might lack in many other people.

The first benefit of this book might be for many millions of people in America and across the world coping with coronavirus, hoping—perhaps against hope—that they and those close to them will survive these hard times. As of this writing, we are still in the middle of the disease outbreak, and its nonmedical impact on people is still to be studied.

What we do know, however, is still cause for concern. By mid-October 2020, over 1,000,000 people worldwide had lost their lives. Millions are infected with the disease, whether they know it or not. Millions more have lost their jobs and incomes. These are all bound to have foreseen and unforeseen consequences and impacts of different types on people. The financial and sociological pressures and problems they are going through are bound to be similar to what I went through. While many undoubtedly will associate with my experiences, many more hopefully will not.

The second type of people who might benefit from this book are the people who are facing hardships unrelated to COVID-19. The number of suicides in the United States alone is unbelievably high and has gone higher since the outbreak of COVID-19.

What you read here might in fact be two separate books. I started writing this long before anyone had heard of the coronavirus. In fact, I had started writing it while I was still going through the hardships you will read later, but I wanted the book to serve a larger purpose. I proceeded to write my chapters to record my experience, but it was my intention from the start to find a way to give it a more expanded perspective. Early in 2020, I decided to renew contact with an old journalist friend who had lost his teenage daughter to suicide. He and his wife had started a suicide public awareness foundation in her memory. I wanted to see if he knew any psychologists or neurologists who might want to partner with me on my project. I wanted someone to read my narrative and then, perhaps, help me with some answers. Was I right in my feelings? Were my reactions either normal or abnormal compared to empirical data or their experiences of other people? How could others benefit from my experiences if they are going through some kind of hardship, showing some of the same symptoms that were visible in me? I wanted the collaborative work to raise further questions and possibly answer some.

So, that is how this book has been organized. As I mentioned, I started writing notes, memos, and thoughts throughout the period of my own struggle. My intent always was to write this book but I put the project aside for various reasons. Back in 2018, I decided to start working on it again, engaged in a lot of research on my own, and turned the material I had into more coherent chapters. I then started collaborating with Jack Lennon, who has considerable background in clinical psychology and neuropsychology. He read my chapters and wrote his own complementary chapters in response to mine. I have revised some of my chapters since, but only in terms of editing and better organizing them; editorially, they are the same as they used to be.

I don't claim that I agree with everything Jack has written, as I suspect he thought some of the ways I had gone about researching my topics were not the best, but he and I are not collaborating on this project so that he would put his stamp of approval on my opinions, or the other way around. The idea is that if there is anyone out there who is going through the same experiences I went through and might be thinking the same things I did, this book might expand his or her horizon by having access to some professional ideas, based on which they could (re)evaluate their own conditions and situations.

Another reason I chose Jack for this collaboration is his approach. In my own research, I found that many of the issues I was grappling with were dealt with in a linear way in the scientific literature, but I was looking for a "Dr. House," someone who would look at symptoms from a multi-disciplinary perspective who would combine psychology, neuropsychology, neurobiology, and cognitive neuroscience all at once to provide a wider analysis. Once you have been able to analyze the problem better, it becomes much easier to deal with it.

For that alone, I thank Jack for his help and insight. His full bio is at the end of this book, as is a brief introduction about me.

Disclaimer:

Introduction

To understand this book better, you need to know more about me, where I came from, how and why I ended up in the United States of America, and how that transplantation shaped me and ultimately contributed to taking perhaps the most potentially consequential decision of my life.

I was born to a middle-class family in Iran. Even in that patriarchal society, my mother was the most educated person in the family. She had a master's degree and was a university professor. My father, far less educated, was what you could call a good technocrat. He was a bank manager and had moved up the ladders to become a regional chief. They and my two other siblings moved every few years from one province to another as he got new assignments. While he respected my mother's educational acumen, she smartly balanced between giving in to his role as the "head of the family" and shaping the family with her intellect.

Neither one was particularly an ambitious person, in the sense that we Americans know ambition as a trait for which you work hard and compete with others, often in a cutthroat environment. My younger brother and sister were blissfully "normal" too, though neither would come close to Michael

Douglas's character in *Wall Street* or Demi Moore's in *GI Jane.*

I, on the other hand, was an abnormal child, much unlike the rest of the family. How, why, or from whom I acquired the genes that differentiated me from the rest of the kettle of fish I do not know. I was born so weak that for the first couple of years of my life our family doctor kept warning my parents that I would probably die soon. I did not die, but I also did not talk. Not a single word came out of my mouth until I was about five years old. I remember the occasion to this day. There was a family gathering at the house of one of my mother's close relatives whose husband was a super-rich businessman. People were talking to each other in the large family dining room on the ground floor. Someone said something, and out of nowhere came a child's response in a near-complete sentence.

That was me. I had finally spoken, and my mother never lets me forget that "to this day we can't get you to shut up!" You could say I have been trying to make up for the lost times ever since.

From the earliest days that I have known myself, I have been a highly ambitious, highly strung person, a sort of Type-A* person who had high dreams for

---

* *Throughout the book, readers would notice that both Jack and I use*

the type of professional and personal goals and lifestyle I have wanted to have, the kind of life no one else in my family had or has. I started working as the host of a children's TV program at the age of nine, even though I was already an active gymnast and member of the chess club. I finished my primary and high school while always having some part-time work and had full-time jobs while going through my undergraduate and graduate schools, both in Washington, DC.

Even before I emigrated to the United States, I knew that I was born in the wrong country. My earliest memory of my infatuation with America was on August 8, 1974. When everyone else in the family was busy with something else, I vividly remember being glued to the radio listening to a rerun of Richard Nixon's resignation speech at the White House, and later watching his famous goodbye gesture as he boarded the helicopter. I was only twelve years old. Even back then, I knew I wanted to be an American, that I mentally belonged to a different place, that one day I would leave the place in which I did not feel totally comfortable but was too young and too immature

---

terms but we might mean different things by them. I have used terms such as "Type A," "Depression" and "Suicidal type" in a non-scientific manner, as one might describe in a daily conversation. Jack speaks of these terms in the scientific fashion, at times providing precise definitions used in clinical and/or research work.

to know why. It was only years later, when I had emigrated to the United States, that I could explain my feelings and convictions in a more formative and educated manner and why, deep down, I subscribed to and valued the socio-cultural, politico-economic principles that came with that faraway continent.

If the seeds of transplantation were with me from an early age, actual life in America gave me roots in a place that has produced a totally different tree, to the point that over the years and decades I have purposefully cut ties to the old place, to the degree that I literally have no ties left and become a full-fledged American, not a hyphenated American.

Maturing as an American helped me to maintain the same Type-A, goal-oriented mentality that says you should expect to know what you want from life, work hard for it, and try to get your dreams materialized, that you don't lower your goals or bring down your standards. You always shoot for higher. You always work to raise the bar, increase the standards. I always have a project. I am always working toward a goal, be that learning a language, writing a new book, or looking for a better-paying job so I have to worry less about retirement.

But achieving the American dream not only is difficult, depending on how much pressure you put on yourself, it also can become quite painful if the dreams do not materialize.

It was the summer of 2015 when a United Nations-associated tribunal in The Hague, Netherlands, asked me to become its head of communications for a temporary period of six months, subject to renewal. I had already gone through a competitive recruitment process for the same position in 2013 when the then incumbent had taken a yearlong leave of absence. For the first six months, they did not hire a replacement. They did so for the second six months on the suspicion that he might not come back. He did. I vacated my post and went to another job in Yemen. By the time I received the call in 2015, the same incumbent had formally resigned, and the tribunal could not wait to advertise the position and go through another round of recruitment, a process that usually takes many months. So, they asked me if I wanted the job for six months. The deal was that they would advertise for the position on a long-term basis after the six months, and I, being an internal candidate, would have a good shot at it.

Those six months were both hard and promising. By December, the tribunal had advertised and shortlisted half a dozen candidates, with me as the only internal candidate. In the end, I did not get the job, not so much because of anything I had or had not done, but because the level of turf battles between my boss and the president of the tribunal was so ferocious that they, and others on the selection committee who sided with one or the other, managed to disagree on every single candidate. For the second time in three years, they showed me the door, this time in perhaps the meanest, least polite, least appreciative manner an employee can be treated.

Just like the millions of people suffering now, I suffered a prolonged period of unemployment, severe physical illness, and crushing mental health pressures. I was a broke, over fifty, white male. The blow was crushing, and I could not handle it any longer.

Having voluntarily and gladly left the place in which I was born for a place for which I had high dreams and in which I had worked hard, the financial hardships that the tribunal experience put me through made me question a lot of things about my life. Sticking to my principle of not lowering my standards, after a year of not having earned a penny, having spent all my savings, taken out every loan I could, I had decided that enough was enough. I was going to take my own life.

Introduction

(By Jack Lennon)

The intention of these comments is to offer a scientific explanation for real-life events, a real journey through difficult times. The goal is to provide relevant references when warranted but not to overwhelm; the information should be easy to understand without being filled with unnecessary jargon. However, readers can review the references (provided at the end of each chapter), should they have interest, thereby increasing their understanding of these topics. Further, looking up the references within these chapters will demonstrate what strong, peer-reviewed articles look like—the types of information that one should rely upon rather than online articles that may unintentionally misinterpret scientific findings.

Risk factors will be an important term to understand. These can be understood as variables that are often found to be related to, or associated with, a particular outcome. They are not required to be present, but in terms of our scientific knowledge, they are often present. This chapter notes at least four major risk factors for depression and suicide, based on the preceding chapter: 1) major life change (losing job); 2) general unemployment/financial instability; 3) reclusive or isolative behavior beyond what is typical for the individual; and 4) male gender.

Unemployment is a serious concern as it relates to suicide, due to the significant financial complications that can stem from it, along with the time-intensive and tedious processes to receive unemployment benefits in certain countries (Blakely et al., 2003). Unemployment is currently at a peak due to the COVID-19 pandemic. Certain studies have found that financial instability is associated with suicidal behavior, such that minimum wage laws can be helpful in confronting this pandemic. For example, one study found that a one-dollar increase in minimum wage resulted in a 3.4 percent decrease in suicide mortality for those with lower educational attainment in the United States (Kaufman, Salas-Hernández, Komro & Livingston 2020). Another study found that, given the known associations, a 1.9 percent reduction would occur following a one dollar increase in minimum wage across the entire population (Gertner et al., 2019).

Social isolation is not only an important sign among those who are depressed and behaving in a manner that is atypical for them, but is a risk factor for suicide (Calati et al., 2019). This can extend to feelings of loneliness as well as the mere act of being alone. Individualistic and collectivistic cultures will differ in this area, but loneliness is generally found to be unhealthy both emotionally and, subsequently, physically (Heu et al., 2018). One can feel lonely in a crowded room, while one can also be content by himself or herself. People are often a combination of characteristics—introverted or extroverted, social or asocial. These are two different dichotomies. Introversion and extroversion are often confused with whether or not someone is social or asocial. These terms actually refer to how one obtains energy—what fuels an individual, being alone or being around others? Therefore, someone can be a social introvert or an asocial extrovert; this is often the case. The degree to which isolation is going to impact someone is related to the basis for it, whether or not someone wants to be isolated, whether or not other stressors are present, and just one's mood in general, but over time, social interaction is helpful to engage in. Again, concerns related to changes in behavior should not be rooted in normative (typical) behavior; it should be based on what is typical for the individual.

Personality types such as A and B are part of a popular hypothesis first noted in the 1950s to describe individuals who are either ambitious, organized, proactive, and perfectionistic or more hedonistic in the sense that they are calm-headed, live with less stress, and do not engage in heavy competition. What must be noted about these personality types is that while they are often used in the English language, they are incredibly vague. There are countless personality features depending on theory of focus. It is easy to describe ourselves as Type A or Type B, which may serve an interpersonal purpose, as well as hold meaning to us internally. However, one should interpret with caution what is stated about these personality types. The components within them, however, are more noteworthy. Perfectionistic tendencies in a reality that all but prohibits perfection can be frustrating. Being highly motivated often leads to rejection in the current academic and vocational climates. Rejection can be met with both positive and negative attitudes, which will vary by person. It is reasonable to suggest, though, that one who is consistently striving for greatness is more likely to experience rejection than a person who approaches life more slowly and takes fewer risks. Much of academic and vocational life is a game of numbers, politics, connections, and luck. Working hard can pay off in the end, whether that be through accomplishing a specific goal or simply through learning important life lessons. Other times, hard work does not result in the achievement of specific goals. The degree to which one is impacted by these outcomes depends on various factors, such that one could certainly become depressed, angry, frustrated, or at least feel understandable sadness.

We may define ourselves however we deem fit. Online tests that claim to ascribe personality traits by asking questions are generally not reliable or valid measures that can be used to draw meaningful conclusions unless they are reputable and affiliated with a university for research or educational purposes. Licensed clinical psychologists are better equipped to do this if one is interested in learning more, as they are trained to administer valid tests that have been tested and are proven to be reliable. These types of diagnostic tests are generally unavailable to the public because their contents cannot be compromised, and they are under copyright. At the same time, one important consideration among all of this is that one should avoid labeling himself or herself to never return to that label. What is meant by this is that life has its peaks and troughs; we change on a molecular level through every interaction, and sometimes these changes are quite remarkable on a behavioral level over time. We are not destined to be anyone; we go through life, and that pathway is what defines us each day. If one is fixated on being a particular person in spite of its consequences or lack of results, it may be worth revisiting the approach, the goal, or the label. One is likely to describe oneself in various ways over a lifetime, and this is merely a process of learning. A person may always have characteristics of the Type A personality, and there is nothing wrong with that unless it begins to create negative consequences. If this happens, evaluate why these events are occurring and alter course accordingly. This does not necessarily entail deviating from goals or dreams, but possibly how one pursues them. If we defined ourselves at eight years of age and never returned to that definition, many of us would be engaged in very different activities right now.

One must be honest and kind to the self. Life is too difficult to approach it any other way.

References

Blakely, T. A., Collings, S. C. D., & Atkinson, J. (2003). Unemployment and suicide: Evidence for a causal association. *Journal of Epidemiology & Community Health, 57,* 594-600. https://doi.org/10.1136/jech.57.8.594

Calati, R., Ferrari, C., Brittner, M., Oasi, O., Olié, E., Carvalho, A. F., & Courtet, P. (2019). Suicidal thoughts and behaviors and social isolation: A narrative review of the literature. *Journal of Affective Disorders, 245,* 653-667. https://doi.org/10.1016/j.jad.2018.11.022

Gertner, A., Rotter, J. S., & Shafer, P. R. (2019). Association between state minimum wages and suicide rates in the U.S. *American Journal of Preventive Medicine, 56*(5), 648-654. https://doi.org/10.1016/j.amepre.2018.12.008

Heu, L. C., van Zomeren, M. & Hansen, N. (2018). Lonely alone or lonely together? A cultural-psychological examination of individualism-collectivism and loneliness in five European countries. *Personality & Social Psychology Bulletin, 45*(5), 780-793. https://doi.org/10.1177/0146167218796793

Kaufman, J. A., Salas-Hernández, L. K., Komro, K. A., & Livingston, M. D. (2020). Effects of increased minimum wages by unemployment rate on suicide in the USA. *Journal of Epidemiology & Community Health, 74,* 219-224. https://doi.org/10.1136/jech-2019-212981

Beginning of the End

Jack Lennon's last sentence in the previous chapter said, "One must be honest and kind to the self. Life is too difficult to approach it any other way." On Thursday, October 20, 2016, I actually was trying to be kind to myself.

It was 5:00 a.m., and I was at my house in the South of France and had woken up just over two hours earlier to watch the third and last round of live debates between the two rivals for the US presidential elections.

I had woken up the same time twice before in the past five weeks to watch the previous two rounds of debates between Hillary Rodham Clinton and Donald J. Trump. Perhaps like millions of other Americans, I was ambivalent about for whom I was going to vote. I pretty much hated Trump and was sure I would not vote for him, but I was equally unimpressed with Clinton and was looking for any and every excuse I could find not to vote for her either.

The last debate, like the two before it, did not persuade me one way or another. Clinton was the same smooth political operator she always was. Trump was the same arrogant and idiotic person millions of Americans had gotten to know the previous year.

So, after watching some of the after-debate political ranting on CNN, I turned off the TV and went to bed. But I could not sleep. I knew what was going on. I had had the same feeling on and off for the past eight months, since January of that year, and for a few months the year before.

I really wanted to sleep. I was tired, both because, well, it was still kind of middle of the night, and because the debate was so uninspiring that I had not really woken up in the first place. but I could not sleep. I kept turning and tossing in bed. The very same thoughts that had engulfed and tired me for months were once again using my head as an unwitting playground. They were not the kinds of thoughts I was willing to accept easily. They were only thoughts of the last resort.

The problem was that I could not deny to myself that the last resort might not become inevitable, even though I was still fairly comfortable that even if I had to succumb to that inevitability, I still had a few months on my hands.

To say that the months between January 2016, when I lost my job at the tribunal in The Hague, and that October morning were hellish is an understatement. Soon after I left the quiet suburb of The Hague, I also fell very sick, which lasted many months. The day-in-and day-out mechanics of finding a new job and the financial impact of not finding one after ten or eleven months were one thing. The anger and frustration over *how* I was let go had built up an intolerable psychological pressure. I was angry when I left and I had remained angry throughout the pursuing months. Even under normal circumstances, my boss was not known for his moral fortitude. He had a reputation inside the building for being indecisive, lacking loyalty, and basically only doing things that would solidify his own position. He was only loyal to himself, even if you had shown loyalty to him in his battles against others, which I had. Even when it had become clear by Christmas 2015 that I would be out the door in three weeks, he made absolutely no attempt to meet with me in person before I left to say thanks or even bye. Human decency was not a quality you would associate with him.

As I sat in bed that early morning and thought about what seemed like my professional and financial end, I also thought about the beginning of my life journey. I wanted to satisfy my own curiosity that I was not folding simply because I was going through a difficult time, even though this was by far the most difficult situation in which I had been. I wanted to remind myself that every difficult situation at the time of its occurrence is just that, a difficult situation. I remembered the time, at the relatively tender age of eighteen, that I covered my first war as a reporter. I had just graduated from high school a few months earlier and was working for an English daily in the capital, Tehran. Not long after the Islamic Revolution in 1979, Iraq invaded Iran. Months later, I was on a government-organized tour for some reporters to the war front. I had mixed feelings. On one hand, I was a teenager with little "action" experience, serious journalism experience. On the other hand, I was a keen and anxious young journalist, wet behind the ears but eager to prove myself and step up the professional ladder.

So, as I sat on my bed, I remembered how we took the local flight to the nearest battle zone city and were then taken by bus to the closest battle area. I had never taken the plane before and remembered being apprehensive, though I am sure I tried to hide it. On the battlefront, we were given helmets but no bulletproof vests. Even the soldiers did not have them. We were told the enemy was on the other side of a hill in front of us. No sooner had we taken cover behind some raised earthen barriers than we heard sounds of artillery and then large puffs of dust from our side of the border. I saw a soldier who gave out a really loud scream not too far in front of me. Not sure why, but I was about to instinctively run towards him when an older and more experienced reporter next to me pulled me down. The soldier in front of me was dead. He was the first dead body I had seen, but I saw many more during my career as a reporter. Needless to say, that day and that image will always remain with me. The colleague who pulled me back probably saved my life, because there were a few more artillery rounds before they stopped. We stayed there for a few hours, although we were pulled back from the frontlines rather quickly. A few commanders were on hand to take some questions, as were some of the soldiers. I remember some of them were not much older than myself back then. By day's end, we were back in the capital and I gave my notes to my editors, who combined them with the day's other war stories. A senior colleague produced the report for next day's front-page story.

Was that a difficult day? A difficult set of circumstances? For an eighteen-year-old, you bet it was. How does it compare to the situation I was in 2016? Obviously, it pales in comparison. But the juxtaposition of the two experiences in my mind served a couple of purposes. First, it was an admission to myself that perhaps after several decades of pushing myself to do better for myself in life, perhaps my "model life" project was not going to happen after all, either because, as in the case of the warzone coverage, I was not experienced enough to know how to meander my way around, or, as in the case of the tribunal, I faced people who were only interested in themselves and were bound by no higher principles.

Meanwhile, I could not forget that the sickness was lingering on, and so did my unemployment, and down went the balance on my bank account. I was broke, had taken every loan I could, and emptied any account I could withdraw from. By the time I reached the early hours of that chilly October morning, I had decided that I might after all have to take my own life around March or April of the following year, by which time I expected I would be totally out of money and have nowhere to turn.

But before that happened, I wanted to write my third book, this one, which back then I thought would be my last one. I had written two novels in previous years, both on current affairs issues that I had turned into fictional stories. Neither one had sold particularly well. The first received different types of criticism, with some of which I totally agree. The second one was better, was written better, and sold more. I enjoy writing novels and decided that should I outlive the crisis on hand and live longer, I would write more. It takes a particular set of skills to write novels, which I did not fully possess when I started writing the first one but started to get the hang of by the time I finished the second. As I mentioned in the prologue, people always told me I should write my memoir, and my answer was always the same: What makes me particular enough to deserve a memoir? I still think I am not special enough to deserve a memoir.

My hardship that year, however, changed my mind. Not because my unemployment and sickness were, *per se*, anything special that would *entitle* me to write a book, but in deciding to commit suicide by a certain time should conditions not change, I had gained new perspectives into and about life that I thought might possibly be of use to other people. I must emphasize that in deciding to pen these pages, there is no intent on my part to teach any lessons or lecture anyone about anything. This is a purely lessons-learned and reflections set of chapters that might—or might not—contain information that would be of use to anyone facing similar hardships. I did not share my intent with too many people, for reasons I will explain in other chapters. But one of the things I learned, and was heartfelt about, was that those friends in whom I confided did not judge me. They did not say, "What a horrible thing to do," "How dare you think so," or things like that. Obviously, they did ask questions like, "Don't you want to live longer?" or "Have you thought how your friends and family will feel?" but those were not condemning statements. They were just trying to see if I had thought things through. And I had, and I responded, and they took my answers at face value.

I also had decided that in the possible likelihood that the book would not be finished by the time I was gone, I would turn over the chapters to my friend, colleague, and established writer and reporter, Janine di Giovanni, and hope that she would finish them for me! Having been a journalist for many years, I obviously know a good many journalists, but Janine is one of the very few who, firstly, is still somewhat in the journalism business and, secondly, had covered many hardship stories and turned them into solid books. I knew, or at least hoped, that she could sympathize and do justice to an unfinished work. Until just a couple of months ago, she never knew about my plans and how I was going to impose on her, but in the end she never had to undergo the burden!

Beginning of the End

(By Jack Lennon)

This chapter is titled as one would expect, such that retrospective reflection often makes the *beginning* of a series of negative events more apparent. This is a highly useful, insightful, and uniquely human ability that should not be taken for granted. We can not only reflect, but we can reflect upon reflection. For example, reflective efforts consider what can be learned from experiences and the value those experiences hold. Analogously, reflexive practice is considering, on a more global scale, the implications of those experiences and learned information specific to the contexts in which they occurred. Depending on the content, it is clear that reflective and reflexive processes can be both positive and negative. What should be avoided is rumination, which is the tendency to dwell on a situation to a degree that negatively impacts one's life, which can be an almost obsessive process for some people if they are very deep thinkers and wish to find clear answers to questions that have no clear answers.

Depression is a term that we all use, often to describe a low mood. We intend no harm, nor do we intentionally use this term to exaggerate a state of emotion. It has, however, found its way into common dialect. Therefore, it is important to distinguish between the two forms: 1) depression as a colloquial way of referring to a mood state at a given time, and 2) clinical depression related to a diagnosable condition (e.g., Major Depressive Disorder [MDD]), which is a cluster of symptoms with specific diagnostic criteria that must be diagnosed by a professional credentialed to do so. The *Diagnostic and Statistical Manual of Mental Disorders* (5th edition), or *DSM-5*, is the classification book for psychiatric disorders (American Psychiatric Association [APA], 2013). The diagnostic criteria allow for some variability in symptoms, such that not everyone will experience MDD in the same way even if the diagnosis is the same. Ultimately, the label is not necessarily that which should be dwelled upon; it is useful for insurance companies and, in some cases, treatment. However, symptoms are often that which are treated rather than the label itself. This is because different symptoms may require different treatments. Thus, whether or not one meets diagnostic criteria for a disorder in the *DSM-5* does not change the reality that he or she is experiencing a specific set of symptoms. The diagnostic criteria for MDD, one of the depressive disorders, is as follows:

"**A.** Five (or more) of the following symptoms have been present during the same 2-week period and represent a change from previous functioning: at least one of the symptoms is either (1) depressed mood or (2) loss of interest or pleasure.
Note: Do not include symptoms that are clearly attributable to another medical condition.

> **1.** Depressed mood most of the day, nearly every day, as indicated by either subjective report (e.g., feels sad, empty, hopeless) or observation made by others (e.g., appears tearful). (**Note:** In children and adolescents, can be irritable mood.)
> **2.** Markedly diminished interest or pleasure in all, or almost all, activities most of the day, nearly every day (as indicated by either subjective account or observation).
> **3.** Significant weight loss when not dieting or weigh gain (e.g., a chance of more than 5% of body weight in a month), or decrease or increase in appetite nearly every day (**Note:** In children, consider failure to make expected weight gain.)
> **4.** Insomnia or hypersomnia nearly every day.
> **5.** Psychomotor agitation or retardation nearly every day (observable by others, not merely subjective feelings of restlessness or being slowed down.
> **6.** Fatigue or loss of energy nearly every day.

7. Feelings of worthlessness or excessive or inappropriate guilt (which may be delusional) nearly every day (not merely self-reproach or guilt about being sick).

8. Diminished ability to think or concentrate, or indecisiveness, nearly every day (either by subjective account or as observed by others).

9. Recurrent thoughts of death (not just fear of dying), recurrent suicidal ideation without a specific plan, or a suicide attempt or a specific plan for committing suicide.

B. The symptoms cause clinically significant distress or impairment in social, occupational, or other important areas of functioning.

C. The episode is not attributable to the physiological effects of a substance or to another medical condition.

Note: Criteria A-C represent a Major Depressive episode.

D. The occurrence of the major depressive episode is not better explained by schizoaffective disorder, schizophrenia, schizophreniform disorder, delusional disorder, or other specified and unspecified schizophrenia spectrum and other psychotic disorders.

E. There has never been a manic episode or a hypomanic episode.

Note: This exclusion does not apply if all of the manic-like or hypomanic-like episodes are substance-induced or are attributable to the physiological effects of another medical condition." (APA, 2013, pp. 160-161).

There is also an exclusion of grief, such that grief differs from a major depressive episode because it will dissipate over time, often in waves, with thoughts about the deceased individual. Preoccupation with a lost loved one is different than the rumination and pessimism found in MDD. Grief can certainly turn into something else over time, but the intention of this note is to ensure that people experiencing completely normative (typical and expected) grief are not unnecessarily diagnosed with MDD. Further, this diagnosis has specifiers including severity, whether or not psychotic features are present, whether or not symptoms have a seasonal pattern, or whether or not anxiety is a prominent feature.

Sleep disturbances (e.g., insomnia, hypersomnia) are heterogeneous (present in many forms based on person) but common experiences for not only people in general but for people at risk for depression. In fact, while the American Psychiatric Association (APA, 2013) describes sleep disturbances as a criterion for MDD, there is evidence to suggest that these sleep issues are more of a predictive sign of depression, though the relationship between the two is complicated (Fang et al., 2019). If one is feeling that sleep is becoming an issue, whether it is too much sleep or not enough, this may be worth reflecting upon. Altering sleep habits is the first step, such as not eating too late, developing a routine, getting out of bed if unable to sleep so that bed is only used to actually sleep, avoid technology prior to sleep, and other strategies that one may consider helpful. Trying to be somewhat active during the day, if possible, may also help with being tired at night while also improving mood. However, these tactics do not work for everyone, so each person will need to consider the degree to which the sleep issues are resulting in negative outcomes in their lives.

It is not uncommon for anger to be a component of depression. This is often viewed as a secondary emotion, such that it can be better described as sadness, disappointment, frustration, or anxiety. However, many certainly experience this as anger toward self or others. Serotonin, a mood-stabilizing neurotransmitter in the brain, is negatively impacted in depression. It has also been found that those with decreased levels of serotonin are more likely to want to punish norm violations than those with typical levels (Enge et al., 2017). This is to say, people with lower serotonin levels are generally more likely to wish to punish those who engage in wrongdoings to a greater degree than those with typical serotonin levels, particularly wrongdoings against the person with low serotonin expression. This suggests that depression, or even a depressive state, could result in consistent and frequent frustration when met with wrongdoings of others. When one is personally attacked or wronged, this is likely to be more pronounced. Further, there is impulsivity that comes from these effects, such that one may act on this anger in some way; this may seem uncontrollable or may even make one feel like they are losing control. When these types of events begin to occur, it is important to consider seeking consultation from professionals to ensure that symptoms do not worsen. One can also work on strategies to overcome these general findings—everyone is different—such that relaxation, breathing techniques, and meditation can be helpful strategies to reduce anger of this kind.

There are two more important comments to make related to this chapter. First, it is not unusual for those who are depressed to consider suicide as an option to avoid or get away from the problems that are resulting in such negative feelings. Some people will make specific plans, some think about it for weeks and others for years. Depending on the person, these plans may be detailed with a very strong intent behind it. Others will consider it a last resort, such that if X does not happen by time Y, then there is always this other option. What one should remember during these times, if this applies, is that there is *hope* involved in this mindset. One has not lost hope but is entirely willing to push through and attempt to accomplish certain goals. This is meaningful. Due to the randomness of life and the amount of luck involved, though, it is important to at least consider what one may feel if the achievement is not met.

The intention to die through a self-inflicted act is a point at which one should certainly seek help from others, if not sooner. This is *not* because these thoughts are wrong—many people wish they had a viable option to live but simply do not see that as an option—but simply because your life is worth living, and there are ways to improve upon some of the aspects people face during these situations. Speaking to close friends can be helpful as well. This chapter describes individuals who were nonjudgmental and caring; these people asked the right questions. If one is fortunate to have these types of trustworthy people in life, it is worth considering discussing with them the suicidal thoughts. This can be very helpful, and one should never underestimate the potential impact of a validating conversation.

References

American Psychiatric Association. (2013). *Diagnostic and statistical manual of mental disorders* (5th ed.). Arlington, VA: American Psychiatric Association.

Enge, S., Mothes, H., Fleischhauer, M., Reif, A., & Strobel, A. (2017). Genetic variation of dopamine and serotonin function modulates the feedback-related negativity during altruistic punishment. *Scientific Reports, 7,* 2996. https://doi.org/10.1038/s41598-017-02594-3

Fang, H., Tu, S., Sheng, J., & Shao, A. (2019). Depression in sleep disturbance: A review on a bidirectional relationship, mechanisms and treatment. *Journal of Cellular & Molecular Medicine, 23*(4), 2324-2332. https://doi.org/10.1111/jcmm.14170

Hope

Hope is important because it can make the present moment less difficult to bear. If we believe that tomorrow will be better, we can bear a hardship today

Vietnamese Clergy Thich Nhat Hanh

I know the book is about a topic that most people find depressing, even me, so I want to start it with an upbeat note about hope. In fact, when I thought every now and then about the possibility of writing a memoir of some sort one day—years and years down the road—I knew what the title would be. I had already decided that I would name the book "*I Believe in a Place Called Hope*" and then write a subtitle underneath saying, "*Yes, I stole it from Bill Clinton.*" After all, if anyone can write one of the most voluminous books of the recent decades, he deserves all the credit he can get!

While the former president was talking about Hope, Arkansas, a place in which he grew up, I am using the word in a more literal sense. From the early days of my childhood, as far back as I can remember, my life was built on hope. I am not sure why I had hope. If Thich Nhat Hanh was right and we have hope for tomorrow because of some hardship today, well, to be honest, I never had what I would consider to be *real* hardship before 2016.

Hope, nevertheless, has been a powerful motive in my life. A clear example was the day that was instrumental in my entering the United States and taking steps towards becoming an American citizen.

On a mild, summer day in 1983, I remember sitting on a bench in the beautiful, green, and well-manicured Giardini di Porta Venezia, an eighteenth-century historic public garden in Milan, Italy. The first bench I sat on was in front of the fountain, next to some of the beautifully arranged flower beds. There were kids running around and making noises. There were also some old ladies sitting on a bench not far away and chatting happily with each other. They were well-dressed and speaking Italian, which I did not understand at the time. I wondered where I would be when I retired and in which shape my life would be. Above all, at that moment I needed peace, even though the sunshine was comforting and making me feel warm, so much so that I took off the leather jacket I was wearing. I contemplated having a drink at the nearby café-restaurant, but I decided to be cheap and not spend the money. So, I walked a bit on the tree-lined pathways and moved to a quieter corner where I could concentrate on why I was there. I had not come to Milan as a tourist. I was scheming, and I needed to get my story right and appear convincing.

If I did not deliver, all hopes would be dashed, hope for a long-standing dream, hope for a better life.

After I had escaped Iran for my reporting in the aftermath of the Islamic Revolution and smugglers took me through a mountainous road to the bordering Pakistan, I finally landed in Beirut, the Paris of the Middle East, the capital of Lebanon. Part of my underground reporting in Iran was for the American news agency The Associated Press during the American hostage crisis, and I hoped the AP would give me a job. I also had been accepted to the American University in Beirut, where I hoped to continue my education. A year after I arrived in Beirut in the summer of 1981, Israel invaded Lebanon, the university closed its doors, and by the following year it had become clear that Lebanon was not a safe place for a young Iranian who did not subscribe to either the revolutionary movements of the clergy or the chaotic politics of Lebanon.

I had to hatch a plan to finally make it to the United States of America. A well-placed and famous Italian journalist friend with connections at the US Consulate in Milan had agreed to help me get an appointment to apply for a tourist visa. The pretense was that I was using the aftermath of the Israeli invasion and the summer vacation to go and see friends in Chicago, who had kindly sent an invitation letter. Between that, my roundtrip ticket in hand, and the recommendation of my Italian friend to his consulate, my friends in Chicago and I hoped the ruse would work and the consulate would buy the story. The plan from the beginning was that I would seek political asylum once I arrived in the States.

As I sat in a quiet and beautiful corner of the park, which has since been renamed to honor an Italian journalist shot by the terrorist group the Red Brigade, I rehearsed my story. I thought about what I might be asked and practiced my answers, trying to look calm but convincing. I was nervous but tried not to think about it. My appointment was in a couple of hours, and I wanted to nail the interview. The interview went smoother and faster than I thought. Mind you, this was the 80s. Getting a US tourist visa these days is a much more Herculean effort! In the end, between hope and practice, I was successful, and I walked out of the consulate with a single-entry tourist visa.

I was beyond happy but, to my own surprise, I was not about to yell and scream in joy or grab the first passerby and give him or her a hug. It was more relief that I was feeling, knowing full well that while

I had a new life in front of me, it was a totally unknown life too.

While that certainly was not the first time I had relied on hope, the Milan experience was a clear reminder to myself of the need for the feeling. Having said that, I have tried not to go down the hope route too far. Truth be told, I have always had a philosophical problem with people who seem to be perpetual "feel good" types, the eternal optimists. To them, everything will always turn out well, that things will always turn out for the best. I find that line of thinking a bit too patronizing and a bit insulting. I think that if you want to be sympathetic with someone who is in trouble, the last thing you want to do is to appear as if you are minimizing the pain and discomfort they are in by simply saying, "Oh, you'll be just fine! Things will work themselves out!" How do you know that? Well, actually, you don't. And you don't know my situation; you don't know why I am where I am. There is a difference between empathy and "Don't worry. You'll be fine."

The other problem I have had with relying too much on the hope factor—much more so lately—is that it seems to me you have to know what you want before you can expect life to work its magic for you. It sounds only fair. You shouldn't ask life to just give you something if you don't have something in mind. That's another problem I have with the concept of Destiny. God (or some other Super Power) has already decided what your fate will be. Okay, why should I bother then if it is all predestined? I don't believe in predestination. I believe in making my own destiny. But generosity should have its limits! I will discuss my past challenges in other places, but for now let's just say that my problem in the past fifteen years or so has been that I have had, or have chosen, to change course in life several times. From that perspective, I have had to be mindful of the fact that it has been hard to ask life to answer my "prayers" if I have not always known what I am asking.

(Disclaimer: One of the recurring lines in this book is "I did not know much about XYZ before I started writing these pages, so I have researched it." Sorry!)

I started doing some research on the question of hope when I started writing this book so I could understand my own actions better. I am sure tens of millions of people, if not hundreds of millions, around the world are resorting to some kind of hopeful thoughts to go through these difficult times of coronavirus. I hope everyone's hope comes true, and I certainly don't mean to question other people's ways of getting through hard times. Maybe some of my ideas and those of Jack Lennon will resonate with people, in which case my wish—and I am sure his—has come true.

One of the people who has done a lot of research on hope and the science of hope is Shane J. Lopez, PhD, who published a book titled *Making Hope Happen: Create the Future You Want for Yourself and Others.* There is a lot about his conclusions with which I disagree, to be frank. Lopez, who is also a Gallup senior scientist, says hope includes anything from joy and awe to sheer excitement but adds that hope is not empty, tunnel-vision optimism. Optimism, he says, is an attitude, while hope is "the golden mean between euphoria and fear. It is a feeling where transcendence meets reason and caution meets passion." You think your future will be better than today. But hope is both the belief in a better future and the action to make it happen. "When hoping," says Lopez, "I felt compelled to act. Hope came along with a whole rush of plans for moving toward the future."

I think I can go along with that distinction, although I would add that, at least in my case, there were a whole lot of other mitigating factors that turned lack of optimism into lack of hope, and therefore the lack of the "rush."

In his book, Lopez says, "How we think about the future—*how we hope*—determines how well we live our lives." In his mind, hope is intricately tied to the future. "I used to think hope was just a warm, vague feeling. It was that sense of excitement that I got before Christmas when I was a child. It lingered a while and then disappeared," he writes. As he develops the theory of the correlation between hope and future, he writes that he became convinced of the interrelations. "I tried not to think about the future. Go ahead, try that for a bit. Unless you are in a deep meditative state, totally focused on a task, or sleeping, your mind goes to the future within minutes, maybe even seconds."

Speaking of a client he was working with, John, Lopez says, "When he had clear hopes for the future, his life was good. When John had a sudden break with his future, he felt his life was not worth living." Judging by his overall experiences, Lopez says, "[O]ur relationship with the future determines how well we live today."

I used to agree with this to a large degree, up until about ten or fifteen years ago. I didn't have that mentality when I was growing up. After I emigrated to the States, the idea of being or becoming "successful" became ingrained in my body and soul—although, as I have said, I was rather goal-oriented from an early age. It was part of my Americanization, part of becoming so competitive in life that it almost necessitated knowing where and what you wanted to be five, ten, or fifteen years down the road. I was exposed to, or exposed myself to, so much talk about long term planning, having five- and ten-year plans for yourself. I was about forty when I realized that my successive plans were not working. That's also when I started changing gears in life so often, changing one career to the next. So when Lopez talks about "our relationship with the future determines how well we live today," I get it. I get it because I was that kid. I also get it because I lived much of my life living hopes that made me stress over life; I get it because, in many ways, I didn't have a life, or at least not one that I enjoyed. That remains the case to today!

I just spent my years trying to bungie jump from one hope to another.

I also mentioned that in my case, there were a whole lot of other mitigating factors that turned lack of optimism into lack of hope. Lopez also addresses the hated F word: Fear! "Hope also walks hand in hand with fear, one of the most universal and most painful emotions. When fear is working for us, it reminds us of the realistic limits or alerts us when we're straying from our path to a meaningful future. But fear can also hijack us. Fear gives us only three behavioral options: fight; flight, or freeze."

There seem to be different types of hoping. Psychologists say people hope, primarily, in two different ways. They hope for "big" things and for "projects."

It might sound strange but, if you think about it, it makes a lot of sense. I don't know about other people but, at least for me, it is easier and more manageable to hope for small things—projects—because I can then point to something tangible in a shorter period of time and actually be happier because I have something to point to. And when you are in trouble in life, when things look really bleak, even small bits of hope matter. Never mind if it actually makes a difference in your life down the road or not. It is not about facts. It is about feelings and emotions. It's about *today*.

Big hopes are life-size or life-duration hopes, say psychologists.

Let me give you a concrete example of a "big idea" type of hope. I have mentioned that I grew up being a journalist, from being the co-anchor of a children's TV program when I was just nine years old, then moving to cover politics and—as the Chinese saying goes—living in interesting times. I covered the Iranian Revolution of 1979–80 and its aftermath, then the Israel invasion of Lebanon in 1982, the Gulf Wars, and on and on till I ended up in Iraq following the 2003 invasion by the United States. So, to say that journalism was and is my first love would not be an overstatement. My big hope was always that I would become some "famous" and "successful" foreign correspondent, like some of journalism heroes of mine. Instead, while I covered some good stories, I was mostly, I never made it to the full-fledged foreign correspondent level. Yes, I have worked for some major hotshot newspapers, news agencies, and broadcast stations like the *Washington Post, Philadelphia Inquirer, San Francisco Chronicle*, Reuters, The Associated Press, Voice of America radio, and Radio Free Europe/Radio Liberty. But, again, most of my journalism career was not on a full-fledged correspondent basis. The big hope is like asking a kid, "What do you want to be when you grow up?" Well, I grew up, but I did not get my first love. To see whether those big picture hopes materialize or not, one would obviously have to wait years, if not decades. In that sense, to have such long-term hopes seems to fall more in the realm of ambition, something you can measure over a much longer period of time.

I think most people would agree that the "magic" of hope works better in the short term. I remember a case in mid-summer 2016, in the middle of my crisis. For months, I had been struggling with what I should do with my house in France should I decide to take my life, keeping in mind that I would only take my life if I totally ran out of money. A little digression here: Under the French law, property goes to the spouse, then children, then parents, then siblings. I am not married, and my parents and siblings would neither have an interest in inheriting the house, nor could they afford the expenses. I consulted a lawyer and went back and forth for months trying to see if I could leave the house for the woman who is my *de-facto* daughter, but she is not legally and formally adopted (because she was too old to be formally adopted by the time she entered my life). So, after many months of researching, consulting lawyers and *notaires* in France, I gave up on the idea and decided to stop spending the money I didn't have on getting her name on the deed. *(Since I wrote this in 2016, France has changed its laws and a non-French resident can designate property by simply stating it in their will, the way I have for my last will in the States.)*

Back to the "small hope" idea and why it matters. As I said, I had been trying for some time to see if there was a way I could lower my expenses so I could live a bit longer. Considering that basically from the beginning of December to more-or-less end of January companies and organizations do not make too many hiring decisions, I figured I would lose those two months trying to find a new job. So, I woke up one morning, making the fate of the house my task to deal with. If I could figure that, perhaps I would wake up less often in the middle of the night out of sheer worry.

My first thought was to sell the house. I even brought in a couple of real estate agents to appraise it, but they said selling the house in a remote part of the country like mine could take six to twelve months. I didn't have enough money to last me six to twelve months, so selling would not have helped, but that morning I came up with two ideas that I thought might actually help. The first was the more unlikely one, but it was worth a try. I have a couple of friends who had talked about the idea of owning a vacation house in the South of France. I was not sure if they would actually like the part of the South of France in which I lived or if they would have liked the house, but it was an idea I was going to try. France also has a system called *Viagé*. It's buying a property based on a long-term agreement with the current owner. The buyer pays a down payment and agrees to monthly payments over a certain period of time, after which the property changes hands. (It's actually more complicated than that, but I am simplifying it here.) That was my first idea for the day, but I must admit that I was not too keen on the idea myself for several reasons. Chief among them was that I went through a lot of trouble to get the house built and for years spent literally all of my spare cash on it. Psychologically, I was just not ready to part with the house, even if I could sell it in the short timeframe I had left and for the amount I liked, which the real estate agents said I could not!

The second thought of the day was much easier to handle. If in the coming months I was still unemployed, it might have made good economic sense to pack everything in the house and just rent it for a year or two until my life sorted itself out a bit. Of course, the downside was that I would most probably have had to spend more cash fixing up the place and repairing whatever damage the renters caused by the time they left.

So, yes, by the time evening came, I was more hopeful. Parenthetically, it turned out many days and weeks later that neither of those two ideas was either a good or a viable one, but as I said earlier, the magic of project-based hope is precisely its short-term impact. It gave me hope that I could kick the can a bit further down the road, and that's what made that day more bearable. I was hopeful that despite what looked like as inevitable—having to take my own life—I might have found a temporary injunction on the continuing life hassles! Did I think my problems were over? Not by a long shot. I am not that naïve. But I realized—and perhaps appreciated—why people believe in taking baby steps and believing in hope in small doses.

Hope

(By Jack Lennon)

Hope is present in ample supply throughout these chapters. It may seem dismal at times, but the willingness and ability to get up and submit job applications, work on that book, read that chapter, make lunch, or make that phone call are all positive signs. This is what is called behavioral activation—doing things that one may not want to do but making an intentional effort to do them anyway. This may seem overly simplistic, but it conditions the brain in such a way that it can prevent a major fallout, depending on one's circumstances. Any reason one can find to engage in a useful or enjoyable activity is a step in a positive direction. Exercise is a heavily supported activity that improves mood in important ways. Even a walk around the block or down the street can be helpful; if you make the walk strenuous enough that you begin breathing heavily, that is even better. At that point, you are providing a service to your heart and your brain.

Many existential questions may arise during times of trouble, as well as perfectly happy times. Those who are highly insightful may see the world in ways that differ from others, which can be both frustrating and disheartening—the world is not necessarily the most pleasant place. How we view these global flaws, however, determines how we approach them and how we feel about our lives. One such question may be related to destiny. Religion has a readily available answer to this question, though many will find that the mystery behind events is difficult to accept. For those who do not align with a particular faith, which is a group growing in size across the world, they may ask different questions. Either way, common questions are those such as "is everything determined in advance?" or "if everything is determined or destined to happen, why even try?" These are deeply introspective questions about life, self, others, and the universe. While no one can provide a verifiable answer with 100-percent certainty, there is something to be said about these questions from a scientific standpoint. Because this topic is not only controversial but quite complicated, we will approach it from a more general and broader lens.

It is true that the physical world—its guiding principles and laws—are deterministic. This is not a hard determinism that would warrant the question "then why try?", because that in itself is a choice. It is a type of determinism that recognizes that every moment is a result of the complex sequence of events leading to it—this is why we behave as we do. There is no logical argument that refutes this reality, albeit a mere fact rather than a comprehensive explanation for any particular outcome. Thus, things are "determined," but destiny has little to do with it from a scientific perspective. At the end of the day, anyone can say that they were destined to be at a particular point, in a particular place, and they cannot be proven wrong. This is not a testable question because we cannot travel back in time and change the life course. It simply is what it is. What we can speculate, though, is that life would likely look different in some way if even one thing from the past was changed. We are all in our current situations because of the complex permutation of events preceding it. Notice that life is not merely a *combination* of events but a *permutation*—the outcome of which depends on the order of events rather than simply the random accumulation of them.

Most importantly, not everyone has the same long list of options at any given time and equal opportunity to choose among them. Here is a salient example: in society, we often view those who commit heinous crimes negatively, which is appropriate, but often for the wrong reasons. It is a fair statement to say that many people believe that the alleged criminal could have chosen otherwise, making people so angry that they seek vengeance in the form of capital punishment in some countries, states, and provinces. Let's look at a very obvious example: an individual with a brain tumor putting pressure on the amygdala has limited choice in emotional reactivity. This individual, from a purely neurological perspective, is going to behave in ways in which he or she otherwise may not. An angry person can engage in behaviors without thinking rationally, depending on the severity of the anger or frustration and its ability to override the rational centers of the brain. The brain chooses responses anywhere from a fraction of a second to seven seconds prior to us being consciously aware of those responses, and we have conducted the functional magnetic resonance imaging (fMRI) studies to prove it. The brain, then, is limited by what it knows to be the best decision for the individual. If one is rational and that has served him or her well, rationality will seem adaptive to the brain. If one has experienced trauma and neglect, very limited education, those options will be far less broad. If one has never experienced love (however one defines it), or experienced love that was combined with violence, that person will learn to behave that way without external assistance or intervention. The apple doesn't fall far from the tree; this is why the cliché sometimes holds true. Imagine being asked to name any country that comes to mind first. There may be a reason you choose a specific country (recently visited, read about, etc.), but not all countries had equal opportunity; there are countries many people have never heard of, thus making those choices literally impossible. The same occurs with behavioral choices. Dr. Sam Harris, a neuroscientist and public speaker, speaks about this topic in the context of morality and often uses similar thought experiments (Harris, 2012).

The one positive component of all this—the *hope*—if it causes concern related to one's own capabilities given the life one has led, is that behaviors are modifiable. This sequence can be altered over the life course, resulting in new behaviors in the future. This is why therapy is helpful for people who need someone to help them develop more efficient steps to getting what they want. Not all therapy is rooted in mere talking. Cognitive-behavioral therapy (CBT) is one that is directive and based on an individual's needs and desires. It focuses on the connection between emotions, thoughts, and behaviors, such that if we alter behaviors, thoughts and emotions can be changed as a result. It eventually entails making small changes to ultimately achieve an end goal. CBT is also the theoretical orientation with the most empirical support for depression. We can engage in new behaviors and think in different ways, which will alter our emotional states and give us new ways of viewing the world, our circumstances, and expand the options available to us (and our brains) at any given moment.

References

Harris, S. (2012). *Free Will*. New York, NY: Free Press.

Suicide

Suicide is the act of intentionally causing one's own death

Stedman's Medical Dictionary

People fear death even more than pain. It's strange that they fear death. Life hurts a lot more than death. At the point of death, the pain is over. Yeah, I guess it is a friend

Jim Morrison

Death is a morbid topic. No one wants to talk about it or think about it, certainly not publicly. I only know of one person who committed suicide. I did not know her well. She was the daughter of the former colleague who helped me find a collaborator for this book and with whom I am happy to be in contact again after many years. But I do know several people who have died of illnesses, mainly cancer, and all of them women. One of them was a very close friend of mine who beat cancer twice but finally succumbed to it. I know of the feeling that the loss of someone you cared about leaves with you. I often think of my friend and miss her greatly. I equally feel guilty that I did not see her during the last few months of her life.

I write these to show that I am not insensitive to the pain that death causes other people, but my own death has never bothered me. It does not mean I wish for it or that I would throw myself in harm's way on purpose. I was certainly close to death during quite a number of assignments I held as a journalist covering wars, revolutions, and uprisings. On several occasions, I found myself in positions that could have cost my life any second. I talked about the first time I was at a war front. The last time I had risked my life was when I was covering the 2003 invasion of Iraq.

One particular date was September 11, 2004. With devastating memories of attacks in the United States on the same day three years earlier still fresh in my mind, I had boarded a small, chartered plane at Baghdad International Airport. Back then, international correspondents covering the invasion would spend six to eight weeks in Iraq and then go back home for a couple of weeks for "rest and recuperation." It was basically to fill out our expense accounts, have a normal life, upload stories and pictures we had not managed to finish, and buy any extra batteries, vitamins, toiletries, or whatever else we could not find in Baghdad. For me, home was Dubai, to which I had moved a year earlier to use it as base just as the world knew we were going to war to topple the regime of Saddam Hussein. I had rented a nice one-bedroom apartment in a decent area of Dubai, though I had spent hardly any time in it up to that point.

On that mid-morning in 2004, about twenty of us boarded the plane. There was still shooting going on around the airport, and the plane was parked as close to the gate as possible. We had waited for a couple of hours inside the terminal, waiting to hear if the flight was go or no-go. Once it was cleared, our passports were quickly stamped, and we made a mad dash to the plane. In less than fifteen minutes, we were all nervously sitting in our seats, security belts tightened, and waited for the luggage to be loaded. After another fifteen minutes or so, the engines started.

The most dangerous part of the flight was still to come. Baghdad airport perimeters were still wide open to multiple militia groups operating in the city. They were all armed to the teeth with rocket-propelled grenades (RPGs), which were unsophisticated and did not have any automatic guiding or heat seeking systems. And the planes on which were flying had no protective defensive systems. In short, the militia groups would simply lob the missiles and our pilots hoped to see them in time to take evasive actions—or not! Sure enough, as soon as the plane took off, I could hear sound of gunfire, which told me someone was firing RPGs. Instead of going the length of the runway to gain maximum speed, the pilots went on a steep climb as soon as they could. There was no word from the cockpit, and the cabin fell into such a deep silence that one could hear if a pin dropped. Within a couple of minutes, the plane was swerving from one side to the other. In a way, that was good news, the pilots had detected the incoming fire and were trying to get the plane out of harm's way. In was not totally good news, because we did not know how many more RPGs were going to target the plane before our altitude would take the plane out of their reach.

A couple of minutes later, the cabin PA system brought the calm voice of the main pilot to us: "We are out of the range." Everyone knew what he meant. Everyone was grateful for their professionalism and gave out a sigh of relief. Soon enough, we were at Queen Alia International Airport in Amman, Jordan, from where we each went our own way.

Obviously, these types of life-imposed deaths threats are very different from intentionally deciding to take your own life. While I had thought about the first type, I had not really given enough thought to the second until my situation in 2016 pushed me that way. (I had toyed with the idea the previous year but it was more on the philosophical level and had not reached the planning level.) It was then that I decided to look more systematically into various aspects of suicide. If you ask "What about it?" I could not answer you. I was not really looking into anything specific, not even how to commit one. I already knew what I needed to do and how to get the material. Perhaps on some sub-conscious level, I was trying to make sense of the decision I had already made and wanted to learn more about myself. Perhaps I would find out more about the thinking, reasons, excuses, and conditions of other people.

Before I get to what I found out, let me address two points that Jack addresses in his chapters. The first is his point about needing to seek professional help when someone was in my situation or if anyone reading these pages is in a similar situation. I would never deny the value of seeking professional mental, psychological, or psychotherapy help. The point I have discussed with him is that when someone like me is already under deep financial and mental pressure, spending time and money to seek professional help is perhaps one of the last things on the list, practically speaking.

That brings me to the second point, which is that in the absence of seeking professional help, one often tries to get as many answers as she or he can on her/his own, which is what I tried to do. But as you will see from Jack's comments, if you are going to do research yourself, you have to ensure that you are thorough. I, especially having been a journalist, tried to be thorough, but I also failed in some instances, as he will point out. So, the importance of finding good information but also doing research on secondary and tertiary sources should not be underestimated.

I must admit that my initial research into the topic of suicide was a bit disappointing because much of the literature I read did not seem to relate to me, my life under the circumstances at the time, what I was thinking, what I was feeling, or anything else. The content in most of the articles I read, scientific or otherwise, could simply be condensed into an online article I found on the website of *Psychology Today* (https://www.psychologytoday.com/intl/blog/happiness-in-world/201004/the-six-reasons-people-attempt-suicide). In it, Dr. Alex Lickerman said there are six reasons people commit suicide:

- **Depression**, which he said was by far the most common reason. "Severe depression is always accompanied by a pervasive sense of suffering as well as the belief that escape from it is hopeless. The pain of existence often becomes too much for severely depressed people to bear."

- **People are psychotic**. "Malevolent inner voices often command self-destruction for unintelligible reasons. Psychosis is much harder to mask than depression, and is arguably even more tragic. The worldwide incidence of schizophrenia is 1% and often strikes otherwise healthy, high-performing individuals, whose lives, though manageable with <u>medication</u>, never fulfill their original promise."

- **People are impulsive**. "Often related to drugs and alcohol, some people become maudlin and impulsively attempt to end their own lives."

- **The person is crying out for help** and doesn't know how else to get it. "These people don't usually want to die but do want to alert those around them that something is seriously wrong."

- **Philosophical desire to die.** "The decision to commit suicide for some is based on a reasoned decision, often motivated by the presence of a painful terminal illness from which little to no hope of reprieve exists. These people aren't depressed, psychotic, maudlin, or crying out for help. They're trying to take control of their destiny and alleviate their own suffering, which usually can only be done in death."

- **They've made a mistake**. "This is a recent, tragic phenomenon in which typically young people flirt with oxygen deprivation for the high it brings and simply go too far."

As interesting as that information was, I am sorry to say that I thought the outlined reasons had little to no relevance to me. I will discuss the depression issue in a little bit, so I am leaving that aside for now. Psychotic? Well, I am sure there are a few people who know me who would say I am psychotic. But seriously speaking, if I were to choose to commit suicide, it was not because some demonic voice inside me was trying to trick me. I do admit that I am often impulsive, but not in the sense that this article was describing. I have never been on drugs, and my alcohol consumption during the crisis since that January had actually gone down tremendously. Crying out for help? That was true in my case, but only in the professional sense, meaning that I have a few people who could have worked harder on my behalf to help me get a job so I could get back up on my feet. Some tried with recommendations, and others networked on my behalf, and I am thankful for that. There are other people whom I wish had helped more actively, but I am not holding a grudge. People don't owe me, so I take what I can! I just wish there was more of it! So, crying out for help? Yes. But not in the emotional sense, which I suppose is what the article was referring to.

But let me go back to the depression part because I think it merits closer dissecting.

To start with, I do admit that I have suspected for years that I have some tiny level of dormant depression in me. It was never a major event. It was not like I would go for days or weeks locking myself up in a room, or hating myself, or needing to consume alcohol on a regular basis to calm my nerves. But this is perhaps a good place to engineer a *mea culpa* section. You see, I have always associated depression with sadness, continuous grief, a state of dysfunction, mental or physical paralysis, or constant demotivation. I have never had those feelings long enough to drive me toward suicide. A few days or a week of sadness or demotivation maybe, but that's been the extent of it. (Sadness is really the only one of the above symptoms I have ever faced, but those were, as I will explain in different chapters, tied to feelings of lack of personal and professional achievement, not anything else.) So, I never considered myself depressed. In fact, the Center for Disease Control in the United States says 7.6 percent of people over the age of twelve have some level of depression in any given two-week period. The World Health Organization goes even further, saying 350 million people worldwide are affected by depression. *(These figures were for the period before COVID-19 started, and I suspect they are higher now.)*

According to the statistics by the American Foundation for Suicide Prevention (https://www.theovernight.org):

- In 2018 (latest available data), there were 48,344 reported suicide deaths.

- A person dies by suicide about every 11.9 minutes in the United States.

- Every day, approximately 121 Americans take their own life.

- There are 3.5 male suicides for every female suicide, but three times as many females as males attempt suicide.

- 494,169 people visited a hospital for injuries due to self-harm, suggesting that approximately twelve people harm themselves for every reported death by suicide.

- Suicide was the second leading cause of death for adults between the ages of 10 and 34 years in the United States.

- Twenty-five million Americans suffer from depression each year.

- Over 50 percent of all people who die by suicide suffer from major depression. If one includes alcoholics who are depressed, this figure rises to over 75 percent.

- Depression affects nearly 5-8 percent of Americans ages eighteen and over in a given year.

- More Americans suffer from depression than coronary heart disease, cancer, and HIV/AIDS.

Did it make me feel better or worse having found out about all those nitty-gritty facts? Not sure, but it did make me more curious.

If depression is supposed to be the leading cause of suicide attempts, I wanted to know more about it. First, I wanted to know what depression is and what causes it. One blog on PsychCentral.com had this useful information on the causes of depression. (https://psychcentral.com/blog/what-drives-a-person-to-suicide/):

"Each of us has swings in our mood or has highs and lows in our emotional feelings. If these swings are within a certain normal range, we remain self-governed and functional. But when they become extreme, they can lead us into the poles of mania and depression. In some cases if the manias become extremely high, the depressions can become extremely low . . . When we are up, manic and elated, our brain can become flooded by increased releasing of dopamine, oxytocin, vasopressin, endorphins, enkephalins, and serotonin. When we are depressed, the reverse can occur, and cortisol, epinephrine and norepinephrine, dihydrotestosterone, substance P, and other neurotransmitters can surge . . . If the manic fantasy becomes extremely high, it can simultaneously be accompanied by a hidden compensatory depression. And if the dopamine rises and we become addicted to our manic states and fantasies, our hidden depressions can grow even more powerful."

There is also lots of literature about different types of depression, none of which applied to me. (Or at least I don't think they did. Could it be that I was just fooling myself? Maybe, but I don't think so. A psychiatrist would perhaps be in a better place to judge this than I am.) The National Institute of Health (NIH) summarized depression fairly well in an online article (https://www.nimh.nih.gov/health/publications/depression/index.shtml):

- **Major depression:** Severe symptoms that interfere with the ability to work, sleep, study, eat, and enjoy life. An episode can occur only once in a person's lifetime, but more often, a person has several episodes. (Of all the types of depression discussed in this publication, this might be the fittest one for me, but I have ruled it out for a primary reason. Depression, I would argue, was not the cause of my not being able to sleep or enjoy life but a symptom; the cause of depression, to the degree that I had any, was my continued unemployment and my perception that that was interrupting my life.)

- **Persistent depressive disorder:** A depressed mood that lasts for at least two years. A person diagnosed with persistent depressive disorder may have episodes of major depression along with periods of less severe symptoms, but symptoms must last for two years.

- Some forms of depression are slightly different, or they may develop under unique circumstances. They include:

- **Psychotic depression,** which occurs when a person has severe depression plus some form of psychosis, such as having disturbing false beliefs or a break with reality (delusions), or hearing or seeing upsetting things that others cannot hear or see (hallucinations).

- **Postpartum depression,** which is much more serious than the "baby blues" that many women experience after giving birth, when hormonal and physical changes and the new responsibility of caring for a newborn can be overwhelming. It is estimated that 10 to 15 percent of women experience postpartum depression after giving birth.

- **Seasonal affective disorder (SAD),** which is characterized by the onset of depression during the winter months, when there is less natural sunlight. The depression generally lifts during spring and summer. SAD may be effectively treated with light therapy, but nearly half of those with SAD do not get better with light therapy alone. Antidepressant medication and psychotherapy can reduce SAD symptoms, either alone or in combination with light therapy.

- **Bipolar disorder** is different from depression. The reason it is included in this list is because someone with bipolar disorder experiences episodes of extreme low moods (depression). But a person with bipolar disorder also experiences extreme high moods (mania).

So far, the literature told me how the brain worked in times of depression, what the symptoms of depression would be and types of depression there were. What I wanted to know was why I would have depression in the first place. Perhaps the next chapter would start to explain that and show some correlation between my life and where I was during my suicidal months.

Despite the high numbers of suicide attempts and completed suicides, there is also a big misconception about the relationship between depression and suicide. Simply put, the general perception is that a much higher number of people try to actually commit suicide than is the case. Depression not only does not directly lead to suicide or attempts to; it is actually a relatively small contributor. Up until a few years ago, it was assumed that up to 15 percent of people "clinically diagnosed" with depression commit suicide. I put clinically diagnosed in quotation marks because actually a small percentage of people with symptoms of depression go as far as seeking professional help—myself included—to see if they qualify for the term or not. Then, the Mayo Clinic in the United States performed a major survey of suicides over a period of thirty years. The November 2000 report put the number of suicides in the United States at 2 to 9 percent, but part of the difference is also due to semantics. Prior to the Mayo research, only people with serious mental illness, like manic depression, were diagnosed with depression. The definition was then expanded considerably to include many other people with mild to serious symptoms of depression that can be treated with therapy or medication. With this broader definition, a much bigger segment of the population can be diagnosed as having depression, and thus the number of suicides count for a small number of people with depression.

In the end—and I am not trying to diminish the importance of the issue at all—to automatically correlate depression and suicide and try to be too rigid about why people get depressed, what kind of depression they have, and then guesstimate what the chances might be that the person might or might not commit suicide really misses the point.

And perhaps even more important than that are the telltales before someone actually does commit suicide. In reality, it doesn't really matter why someone ultimately decides to take his or her life. It matters that they do. I know firsthand of many cases in which people had actually no idea someone was about to commit suicide. But equally, there are plenty of cases in which people around the person simply did not pay enough attention to *see* the signs. When someone suddenly disappears from the "radar" or becomes unusually inward or isolate themselves more than usual and for longer periods than normal, those should ring alarm bells for people around them. It is true that the nature of life has changed in the past decades. Life has become faster, people are busier than they used to be, and the professional world has become more specialized so people have to work harder and longer hours to maintain their job, if not thrive in it, leaving less time for personal life. All of that is true, but none of it is good enough an excuse to take our eyes off danger signs around us.

I am an example of that. Maybe a rare example, but one nevertheless. In my case, I was not planning on committing suicide because I had fallen into a gradual and temporary depression. The depression was occasional, though its degree went up and down at times. I was planning to commit suicide because I had dreams for myself and my life, and I was seeing them being destroyed with no apparent solution before me. And I was there because two idiotic, irresponsible, incompetent individuals with no apparent sense of morality or human decency had all of a sudden pulled the plug on my professional life because they wanted to engage in a bureaucratic turf battle with each other. Those were the two bosses at my previous job before I went through the 2016 year-long unemployment.

Because of that experience, I basically went through a roller-coaster situation in which, on one hand, I withdrew from the world and, on the other hand, craved for company and friendship. Because of where I was living at the time—in a small village in France—the withdrawal part was easy. However, partly because I was living in a remote area and partly because even my close friends were not paying attention to my dilemma, the craving for company and friends was left totally unanswered. With the exception of two or three people, no one noticed that I had stopped communicating, that I was not calling or emailing. Everyone was busy with their life. People were not reading the tea leaves. That in turn multiplied the pressure. Did that cause the depression? No! Did it exacerbate the pressure—I still refuse to call it depression—yes, no doubt. Did it in any way contribute to the decision to take my own life? Absolutely not.

There are two other points that I think need to be discussed in the context of suicide.

The first is that, as I alluded to partially, the formal discussions of the topic of suicide deal more with what I would call the final steps before the actual act. They don't deal as much with the underlying socio-economic causes. They only look at the last chapter of one's life from a medical perspective and then try to add psychological interpretation to explain it. They don't go deep enough. One could argue that perhaps there are too many potential underlying causes and at some point they need to be pushed up into a pyramid format. True, but that is not a good excuse. Again, taking from my own experience and perspective, one of the underlying factors was the sheer sense of frustration, which I would admit could lead most people into depression. For me, and to tie it to another issue of which I have spoken, it is my personal inability to achieve the goals I set for my own life, the lack of realization of which increased my own sense of not being a fully-contributing person in life, and achieving my own personal apex.

The other point, I am sure, will be controversial with many, but bear with me. Suicide is generally seen in most, if not all, societies as something negative, something that should be avoided at all costs. I would argue that some exceptions to that rule might be worth considering. The arguments against committing suicide generally fall into two categories. The first is that life is precious, whether you take that from a religious or civic perspective, and what seems to be an impasse in life will likely get better if you persevere and give it more time. The second argument is that committing such an act will temporarily or permanently shatter the lives and well-being of those around the person who made a decision to end his or her life. On the first point, especially if we take it from the perspective of the person who is in pain, there is no guarantee things will get better. That ties to the second point. Yes, life is precious, but the person should be the owner of the power to make the decision what to do with it, especially if A) you don't have any immediate and particular responsibilities to others like your spouse, partner, children, etc., or B) you have carved a certain life standards for yourself and are not willing to compromise any significant downgrades to that vision. These could sound totally unreasonable and hypocritic arguments, but we need to accept the fact that if a person is really determined to take his or her life, perhaps that is the right decision for them.

At the end of the day, suicide is and should remain a personal decision. And perhaps cutting the stigma out of the discussions about suicide and depression might open the doors for discussing it from other perspectives as well.

A final note on suicide. While I would like to think that I thought rationally about my decision whether to commit suicide or not and analyzed the situation the best way I could, given my own particular circumstances, there is one down side with my own thinking, and I acknowledge it. The problem is that once you open up the suicide can of worms, I am not sure you can safely put the genie back in the bottle. If I get into trouble again, would I be able to stop myself? Would I even be able to maintain what I think was a rational process the first time around? Would I be able to maintain the same level of thought process?

Honestly, I am not sure!

Suicide

(By Jack Lennon)

It is not uncommon for individuals experiencing difficulties in life to seek information, whether it be for pure knowledge and understanding or to feel less alone and more understood. The concern with this quest is the type of information available on the worldwide web. Specifically, the inaccurate information posted, even if unintentional. The intention here is to ensure that everyone can read an article and determine its credibility, which is not always an easy task. However, there are giveaways that can help people better prepare themselves for determining the value of a given article. Further, it is important to help people understand why they may not relate to some of the information that they read, particularly in the context of depression and suicidal thoughts. Some people are able to relate while others do not, and for understandable reasons—human beings are incredibly complex and unique. This is not to say that we cannot understand them, because we understand plenty, but making global statements that will relate to an entire group of unique people is difficult to accomplish when discussing this subject. Further, our diagnostic classification system is based on empirically supported qualitative criteria that both the healthy and unhealthy may experience. When cultural and psychosocial considerations are incorporated, people will experience these symptoms in different ways, which is why it is important to seek professional help so you can be understood in the context of your circumstances.

Understandably, not everyone experiencing minor psychiatric symptoms requires treatment. Not everyone can afford treatment; not everyone has healthcare. This is completely understandable, and in many cases treatment is the last thing people are thinking about. At the same time, if it is at all possible, it is better to receive assistance early before the opportunity is lost to worsening symptoms. It is my ethical duty to state that an expert opinion is the best course of action because they can understand your medical and psychiatric history, should the means be available. One is not obligated to continue beyond that initial opinion, but only a professional can accurately determine what treatments, if any, a given person may benefit from. Serious psychiatric symptoms can stem from various systems in the body, including the endocrine system, such that answers cannot be resolved alone any better than other medical conditions.

I must concede to the fact that the referenced *Psychology Today* opinion article (not a study) was published in 2010, at which time we knew even less about suicide than we do today (Lickerman, 2010). However, given that times have changed, there are several flaws that are important to highlight. In fact, there are flaws that should be noted even if we had not learned anything new over the past decade. This is the issue one will face, though, when researching complex topics such as suicide—we know a lot, but we are confronting a point at which it is difficult to translate information we know about the brain into actionable interventions that can be used for people in need. We have certainly come a long way in terms of psychiatric and psychological treatments, and as suicide rates continue to rise, we are paying closer attention to these risks in patients with risk factors. Unfortunately, risk factors are simply signs that warrant further investigation; they need not be present for an individual to engage in suicidal behaviors, but in many cases at least some risk factors are.

First, we must arm ourselves with knowledge about how to read articles that are not part of actual empirical studies. "Cause" is a very strong word, and it holds substantial meaning in the process of science. Be skeptical of articles that claim causality, and dig deeper if you see this word in relation to psychiatric conditions. Also, when a professional's personal experiences are used to draw conclusions about the general population, consider moving away from that article. One's experiences are not a representative sample of the population, such that any conclusions drawn cannot be generalized to the population. This is what we call external validity, being able to take results from studies and generalize them to other people outside of the study. We actually do *not* know the cause of suicide; we know many risk factors for suicide extending from observable, everyday phenomena to brain changes only visible with advanced technology. We do not know the reasons why any particular individual died by suicide. This is often the most difficult reality for affected families and friends, who often report the individual seeming fine. They will often reflect and recognize signs that seemed trivial at the time, such as social isolation or giving away belongings (Ahmadpanah et al., 2017), but this is merely hindsight combined with a deep desire to answer a complicated question. Therefore, consider searching for peer-reviewed articles, which are less likely to exaggerate interpretations or overstate arguments. If an article mentions a study, search for that study; it is not uncommon for popular media outlets to misunderstand or misstate a study's findings.

Suicide likely *is* more understandable than many believe, despite the belief some harbor that it is too complicated to predict in advance; this is why we study it. Unfortunately, the reality is that clinical accuracy is similar to flipping a coin, even once we better understand the patient (Nock et al., 2010). Some studies have already proven that future suicide attempts are predictable in the populations they were studying. However, the ability to predict in a meaningful way in clinical settings is complicated because we cannot utilize the research measures noted above with all individuals and expect to avoid false-negative results in the population at-large. Hence, this translation to overarching prediction is not as simple as we would like to think it is. As with any field, the more one understands suicide from molecular, physiological, and behavioral domains, the more one realizes that he or she knows very little. Question those who claim to know too much.

The Interpersonal-Psychological Theory of Suicide (Joiner, 2007; Van Orden et al., 2010) is currently a strong basis for understanding suicide from a psychosocial perspective. This theory suggests that two states of being are required to engage in a suicidal act: 1) thwarted belongingness, and 2) perceived burdensomeness. These states must be met with a strong sense of fearlessness, a degree of conviction and focus that is known to significantly reduce one's blink rate prior to a suicide attempt (Joiner et al., 2016). It is of little surprise that depression would be a major risk factor for suicide given this theory, as well as what Major Depressive Disorder (MDD) entails. However, a key point is that depression does not need to be present or diagnosed for an individual to attempt suicide. Most people who are diagnosed with MDD do not attempt suicide.

With that being said, depression is most appropriately described as a risk factor; it is not everyone's reason, and depression is arguably not the underlying reason for anyone. The reality is that we often assume that a suicide death is evidence of depression rather than a discrete trajectory or diagnosis in and of itself (Sisti et al., 2020). We know that significant differences are found within the brains of depressed individuals who do and do not attempt suicide. Further, those who attempt and survive are different than those who die by suicide. These are unique groups of people, and we are not entirely sure why from a clinical perspective, but we do know that the serotonin system, one known for mood stabilization, is a major distinction among these groups (Gould et al., 2017; Underwood et al., 2018). The overarching way to distinguish between sadness or a depressed mood and MDD is the ability to bounce back after a reasonable amount of time. MDD requires a span of ongoing symptoms (several of them) for two weeks or longer, which is why not everyone who is depressed in a general sense may meet criteria for MDD at any given moment.

Psychosis is not generally associated with suicide, though it warrants further investigation from a clinical perspective if one is actively or even passively suicidal. This term is vague, though, as it encompasses several disorders, with schizophrenia being only one of them. Suicide rates in schizophrenia are often found to be fairly similar to those of adolescents and other high-risk groups, but no greater; this risk is skewed and exaggerated because the onset is generally preceded by a higher risk (Brucato et al., 2019). It is important to dissect the noted concerns with "people are psychotic" though. The psychotic feature can be a part of depression, particularly when it is left untreated. This is not a distinct diagnosis but an MDD specifier (APA, 2013). Auditory hallucinations, though, come in a variety of forms, one of which is command-type, which would entail that a voice or voices are commanding the individual to engage in a certain act. These types of auditory hallucinations are uncommon. Secondly, command-type hallucinations that command harm to the individual are even less common; this is more of a Hollywood and media version of Schizophrenia.

This certainly occurs, and there is a reason why we have specifiers with this diagnosis (APA, 2013), but, broadly speaking, they are not generally what we find on a larger scale.

Arguably the most important and common misunderstanding related to suicide is that of impulsivity. From a neuropsychological perspective, this is frontal lobe dysfunction that results in an inability to inhibit behaviors—one cannot suppress his or her impulses (Lezak et al., 2012). It is understandable that people would suspect that suicide could be impulsive, but this has been disproven to such a degree that the misconception must be actively confronted and ameliorated (May & Klonsky, 2016). Suicide is a specific behavior that requires several cognitive faculties to be intact, and this includes executive functions that are located in the frontal lobes and prefrontal cortex. Planning, organization, and task-shifting are all part of this equation. Not everyone who dies by suicide develops a detailed plan, but many do. In Japan, note-leaving generally remains steady at 23.4 to 36.2 percent of suicide deaths even during times of increased suicide deaths (Shiori et al., 2005). Not everyone will follow that plan perfectly, but this is not impulsive in the scientific sense. Most individuals who die by suicide have thought about it for quite some time—anywhere from weeks to several years. As previously noted, individuals on the brink of attempting suicide are highly focused and set in their train of thought—they are not impulsive. If we look at a disorder that is specifically characterized by impulsivity, such as Attention-Deficit/Hyperactivity Disorder (ADHD) Hyperactive/Impulsive or Combined types (APA, 2013), we do not find higher rates of suicide than we do in the general public.

The idea that suicidal individuals are crying out for help is not necessarily inaccurate in all cases, though I disagree with the phrasing. Depending on an individual's circumstances, it is entirely possible and true that some do not want to end their own lives but engage in nonlethal or less-lethal means, such as consuming a large number of pills or making superficial cuts. The latter is what we consider non-suicidal self-injury (NSSI) if the individual reports that there was no *intent*. One's intentions are difficult to determine, but we generally rely on standardized interviews and self-reports to determine this. It is reasonable to suspect that those who are experiencing other difficulties and cannot seem to obtain attention or support may seek it through unsafe means. People have a tendency of engaging in a wide range of behaviors to gain attention, and much of this is based on how we learn to gain that attention over the course of life. The key point here is that attention is not the sole basis for engaging in NSSI or suicide attempts; there is more to the story. One example is that NSSI combined with a history of suicide attempts suggests a greater risk of future suicide attempts than individuals with attempts but no NSSI history (Brausch et al., 2016).

A philosophical desire to end one's own life is a difficult concept to confront simply because of its vague and unclear nature. Those who are terminally-ill or have neurologic conditions, ranging from early Alzheimer's disease (AD; Serafini et al., 2016) to Parkinson's disease (Giannini et al., 2019), Huntington's disease (Kachian et al., 2019), traumatic brain injury (Madsen et al., 2018), and stroke (Bartoli et al., 2017) are at increased risk of suicide. As the referenced article notes, it is more likely that they are more "reasoned," but this merely repeats that which has already been stated above—impulsivity is not the issue here. Depression is also common among these populations, with depression being thought of as one of the first observable signs of AD (Gallagher et al., 2018). The neurodegeneration impacts important brain circuits in areas highly innervated, such as the limbic system, which primarily deals with emotions. As AD progresses, certain faculties are lost that actually reduce risk of suicide—planning, organization, working and prospective memory, among others. Medical conditions such as diabetes and cardiovascular disease are also risk factors (Drapeau & McIntosh, 2020), likely due to the prognoses, and are even more concerning when individuals have limited social support. As you may be noticing, there is a theme here—it is a complex combination of variables that are interrelated. Most people with terminal illnesses do not die by suicide even though euthanasia, or physician-assisted suicide, is becoming more common for those who have been determined to have less than six months to live.

Mistakes do happen. As we currently define suicide in the field, *intent* is an important concept. We can only assume whether or not one intended to end his or her life, though we have psychological autopsies that can try to ascertain the nature of the behaviors (Nock et al., 2017). NSSI, for example, is a risk factor but neither a cause nor a reason for suicide (Burke et al., 2016). At times, NSSI is accidentally more severe than intended. We know that this increases risk of suicide through desensitization, and the fact that those who make these errors are more likely to report intent than those who do not. However, if the individual survives a very deep cut that was accidental and reports that it was unintentional, it would not be considered a suicide attempt; it would be considered NSSI requiring hospitalization. The oxygen deprivation noted in the article follows suit—asphyxiation is an uncommon cause of suicide death, at least in the United States (Drapeau & McIntosh, 2020), unless one is referring to hanging, in which case this is less likely to be one trying to "flirt" with his or her life. As always, though, this is case-dependent. Once a person has passed away, we can only learn so much about the state of mind or intentions. We often assume suicide, but if it truly was an accident as the article noted, this would not be a suicide but instead an accidental death, another very common cause of death in the United States. Oxygen deprivation is more likely to result in other issues, as the brain requires a constant and steady supply, otherwise it can experience irreparable damage.

When one begins to stumble onto discussions related to mania and hypomania, they have likely confronted discussions related to bipolar I or II disorders. It is not uncommon for individuals with MDD to experience mood swings or moments of energy and more uplifting feelings, which we call euthymia (Szmulewicz et al., 2017). It is at these times when an individual is at greater risk for suicide, if he or she was suicidal, because the energy to engage in the act is now available. However, these upbeat moments do not meet the diagnostic criteria for manic or hypomanic episodes in depression unless one is referring to Bipolar Disorder. Manic episodes are characterized by extended periods of time during which there is an uncharacteristically high level of energy, decreased need for sleep, grandiose plans or ideas, increase in risk-taking behaviors including sexual activity, gambling, spending, or other activities (APA, 2013). The two poles refer to the mania and depression, though these generally do not change rapidly within a day; these phases are more spread out in most cases. Mere changes in mood throughout the day can be present in otherwise healthy individuals, and bipolar disorder does *not* refer to those who are happy at one moment and then suddenly become angry seemingly without reason.

Unfortunately, suicide is at an all-time high in the United States—the tenth-leading cause of death—and has been a global pandemic for decades (Drapeau & McIntosh, 2020). We currently lack sufficient primary prevention methods which aim to modify risk factors—socioeconomic status, social class, unemployment, systemic racism, rural living—but these are not readily prepared for alterations on a large scale. Instead, we should be aiming at better understanding the unique combination of factors that suggest one will or will not engage in a suicide attempt, and then what to do to ensure that the individual does not do so moving forward. We know that many people who die by suicide visit a healthcare professional within approximately one month to a year prior to death (McDowell et al., 2011; Raue et al., 2014). This is typically a primary care physician for an unrelated complaint. With sufficient screening and better measures to target suicide risk that may be just as much unconscious as it is conscious, these individuals could receive appropriate treatment before symptoms increase in severity.

References

Ahmadpanah, M., Astinsadaf, S., Akhondi, A., Haghighi, M., Bahmani, D. S., Nazaribadie, M., Jahangard, L., Holsboer-Trachsler, E., & Brand, S. (2017). Early maladaptive schemas of emotional deprivation, social isolation, shame, and abandonment are related to a history of suicide attempts among patients with major depressive disorder. *Comprehensive Psychiatry, 77*, 71-79. https://doi.org/10.1016/j.comppsych.2017.05.008

American Psychiatric Association. (2013). *Diagnostic and statistical manual of mental disorders* (5th ed.). Arlington, VA: American Psychiatric Association.

Bartoli, F., Pompili, M., Lillia, N., Crocamo, C., Salemi, G., Clerici, M., & Carrà, G. (2017). Rates and correlates of suicidal ideation among stroke survivors: A meta-analysis. *Neurology, Neurosurgery & Psychiatry, 88*(6), 498-504.

Brausch, A. M., Williams, A. G., & Cox, E. M. (2016). Examining intent to die and methods for nonsuicidal self-injury and suicide attempts. *Suicide & Life-Threatening Behavior, 46*(6), 737-744). https://doi.org/10.1111/sltb.12262

Brucato, G., Appelbaum, P. S., Masucci, M. D., Rolin, S., Wall, M. W., Levin, M., & Girgis, R. R. (2019). Prevalence and phenomenology of violent ideation and behavior among 200 young people at clinical high-risk for psychosis: An emerging model of violence and psychotic illness. *Neuropsychopharmacology, 44,* 907-914. https://doi.org/10.1038/s41386-018-0304-5

Burke, T. A., Hamilton, J. L., Cohen, J. N., Stange, J. P., & Alloy, L. B. (2016). Identifying a physical indicator of suicide risk: Non-suicidal self-injury scars predict suicidal ideation and suicide attempts. *Comprehensive Psychiatry, 65,* 79-87. https://doi.org/10.1016/j.comppsych.2015.10.008

Drapeau, C. W., & McIntosh, J. L. (2020). *U.S.A. suicide: 2018 official final data.* Washington, DC: American Association of Suicidology. Retrieved from https://suicidology.org/wp-content/uploads/2020/02/2018datapgsv2_Final.pdf

Gallagher, D., Kiss, A., Lanctot, K., & Herrmann, N. (2018). Depression and risk of Alzheimer dementia:

A longitudinal analysis to determine predictors of increased risk among older adults with depression. *American Journal of Geriatric Psychiatry, 26*(8), 819-827. https://doi.org/10.1016/j.jagp.2018.05.002

Giannini, G., Francois, M., Lhommée, E., Polosan, M., Schmitt, E., Fraix, V.,Castrioto, A., Ardouin, C., Bichon, A., Pollak, P., Benabid, A. -L., Seigneuret, E., Chabardes, S., Wack, M., Krack, P., & Moro, E. (2019). Suicide and suicide attempts after subthalamic nucleus stimulation in Parkinson disease. *Neurology, 93*(1). https://doi.org/10.1212/WNL.0000000000007665

Glenn, J. J., Werntz, A. J., Slama, S. J. K., Steinman, S. A., Teachman, B. A., & Nock, M. K. (2017). Suicide and self-injury-related implicit cognition: A large-scale examination and replication. *Journal of Abnormal Psychology, 126*(2), 199-211. https://doi.org/10.1037/abn0000230

Gould, T. D., Georgiou, P., Brenner, L. A., Brundin, L., Can, A., Courtet, P., Donaldson, Z. R., Dwivedi, Y., Guillaume, S., Gottesman, I. I., Kanekar, S., Lowry, C. A., Renshaw, P. F., Rujescu, D., Smith, E. G., Turecki, G., Zanos, P., Zarate Jr., C. A., Zunszain, P. A., & Postolache, T. T. (2017). Animal models to improve our understanding and treatment of suicidal behavior. *Translational Psychiatry, 7,* e1092. https://doi.org/10.1038/tp.2017.50

Joiner, T. E. (2007). *Why people die by suicide*. Cambridge, MA: Harvard University Press.

Joiner, T. E., Hom, M. A., Rogers, M. L., Chu, C., Stanley, I. H., Wynn, G. H., & Gutierrez, P. (2016). Staring down death: Is abnormally slow blink rate a clinically useful indicator of acute suicide risk? *Crisis, 37*(3), 212-217. https://doi.org/10.1027/0227-5910/a00036

Kachian, Z. R., Cohen-Zimmerman, S., Bega, D., Gordon, B., & Grafman, J. (2019). Suicidal ideation and behavior in Huntington's disease: Systematic review and recommendations. *Journal of Affective Disorders, 250*, 319-329. https://doi.org/10.1016/j.jad.2019.03.043

Lezak, M. D., Howieson, D. B., Bigler, E. D., & Tranel, D. (2012). *Neuropsychological assessment* (5th ed.). New York, NY: Oxford University Press.

Lickerman, A. (2010). The six reasons people attempt suicide. *Psychology Today*. Retrieved from https://www.psychologytoday.com/intl/blog/happiness-in-world/201004/the-six-reasons-people-attempt-suicide

Madsen, T., Erlangsen, A., Orlovska, S., Mofaddy, R., Nordentoft, M., & Benros, M. E. (2018). Association between traumatic brain injury and risk of suicide. *JAMA, 320*(6), 580-588. https://doi.org/10.1001/jama.2018.10211

May, A. M., & Klonsky, E. D. (2016). Impulsive' suicide attempts: What do we really mean? *Personality Disorders: Theory, Research, & Treatment, 7*(3), 293-302. https://doi.org/10.1037/per0000160

McDowell, A. K., Lineberry, T. W., & Bostwick, J. M. (2011). Practical suicide-risk management for the busy primary care physician. *Mayo Clinic Proceedings, 86*(8), 792-800. https://doi.org/10.4065/mcp.2011.0076

Nock, M. K., Dempsey, C. L., Aliaga, P. A., Brent, D. A., Heeringa, S. G., Kessler, R. C., Stein, M. B., Ursano, R. J., & Benedek, D. (2017). Psychological autopsy study comparing suicide decedents, suicide ideators, and propensity score matched controls: Results from the study to assess risk and resilience in service members (Army STARRS). *Psychological Medicine, 47*(15), 2663-2674. https://doi.org/10.1017/S0033291717001179

Nock, M. K., Park, J. M., Finn, C. T., Deliberto, T. L., Dour, H. J., & Banaji, M. R. (2010). Measuring the suicidal mind: Implicit cognition predicts suicidal behavior. *Psychological Science, 21*(4), 511-517. https://doi.org/10.1177/0956797610364762

Raue, P. J., Ghesquiere, A. R., & Bruce, M. L. (2014). Suicide risk in primary care: Identification and management in older adults. *Current Psychiatry*

Reports, 16(9), 466. https://doi.org/10.1007/s11920-014-0466-8

Serafini, G., Calcagno, P., Lester, D., Girardi, P., Amore, M., & Pompili, M. (2016). Suicide risk in Alzheimer's disease: A systematic review. *Current Alzheimer Research, 13*(10), 1083-1099.

Shiori, T., Nishimura, A. Akazawa, K., Abe, R., Nushida, H., Ueno, Y., Kojika-Maruyama, M., & Someya, T. (2005). Incidence of note-leaving remains constant despite increasing suicide rates. *Psychiatry & Clinical Neuroscience, 59*(2), 226-228. https://doi.org/10.1111/j.1440-1819.2005.01364.x

Sisti, D., Mann, J. J., & Oquendo, M. A. (2020). Toward a distinct mental disorder–suicidal behavior. *JAMA Psychiatry*. Advance online publication. https://doi.org/10.1001/jamapsychiatry.2020.0111

Szmulewicz, A. G., Valerio, M. P., Smith, J. M., Samamé, C., Martino, D. J., & Strejilevich, S. A. (2017). Neuropsychological profiles of major depressive disorder and bipolar disorder during euthymia: A systematic literature review of comparative studies. *Psychiatry Research, 248,* 127-133. https://doi.org/10.1016/j.psychres.2016.12.03

Underwood, M. D., Kassir, S. A., Bakalian, M. J., Galfalvy, H., Dwork, A. J., Mann, J. J., & Arango, V.

(2018). Serotonin receptors and suicide, major depression, alcohol use disorder and reported early life adversity. *Translational Psychiatry, 8,* 279. https://doi.org/10.1038/s41398-018-0309-1

Van Orden, K. A., Witte, T. K., Cukrowicz, K. C., Braithwaite, S. R., Selby, E. A., & Joiner, T. E. (2010). The interpersonal theory of suicide. *Psychological Review, 117*(2), 575-600. https://doi.org/10.1037/a0018697

Mentors

We are the victims of our ow anxieties

Israeli author and psychologist Ayelet Gundar-Goshen

A lie is more comfortable than doubt, more useful than love, more lasting than truth

Gabriel García Márquez

A picture and a hug would best summarize the next few pages, but the experiences behind them mean so much more to me. So much so that I am sure my limited writing skills will fail to explain adequately. Here is an attempt anyway.

Neither of the two people referenced in this chapter know that I am mentioning them—or, for that matter, that I am even writing this book.

Right before I started this chapter, I once again looked at a picture of the first person I consider a mentor. He had posted the picture of himself on a social media page a while back entering the White House Oval Office as he accompanied a former United Nations secretary-general for a meeting with the then-president of the United States. Standing tall and slim in a nice suit next to the US president, the person I am calling *A* is someone I have dreamed of being, not literally of course! I try to be a reasonable in life, so I would never dream of being as smart as him, or as tall and distinguished looking as him! He was born into a life of intellectual privilege. My family was an ordinary middle class one, and if I become half as educated and informed as he is, I would be pretty happy with myself. After spending more than twenty years working for the United Nations in various capacities and in various parts of the world, he rose to one of the highest positions, before choosing to leave the UN and put his vast skills to other use. He works incredibly hard and is incredibly kind.

I said this chapter is symbolized by a picture and a hug. The hug part is about an encounter with a person I call Z, another mentor of mine in the UN system. Z was once my supervisor. We both went through a difficult period at the place we worked. She was, and is, much more superior to me in rank and achievements in the UN system and life as a whole. I have always admired her not only for the fact that she has shot up in ranks, but I also respect her for the way she has done it. She has worked in god-awful countries under god-awful bosses, but she is politically savvy enough and mentally strong enough that she has survived the "system" and managed to thrive in it—and done all of that knowing that she too will leave the UN one day and then do the things she really wants to do. She, too, is an embodiment of who I wanted to be. For those reasons, plus the fact that she has always been a good friend to me, I think the world of her and have yearned for her reciprocal respect, fully realizing that I have not earned it—yet. I continue to limp along while she keeps going up the ladder rungs.

Late in 2017, after I had gained some temporary work and was off my self-enforced suicide track, I had an opportunity to walk into Z's office. We had not seen each other for a few years, though we had remained in touch throughout the time, and I benefitted from her advice and wisdom when I could. The second I walked into her office, she walked over from her desk and gave me the warmest and most sincere hug I had received for I don't know how long. Even now, a couple of years after that encounter, I remember the warmth, sincerity, and genuineness of her embrace. I remember I was literally fractions of a second away from breaking into tears and throwing myself into her arms again. It was a short few months after when I thought I would be dead—though she had no way of knowing it—and the fact that my dear former boss and mentor was giving me a hug was validating my existence—almost literally—and reinforcing why she is my mentor.

Why do I say *A* and *Z* are embodiments of who I *wanted* to be? Why do I put it in the past tense? Because I know I cannot and will not be able to achieve what they have achieved. I have reached an age where moving up the corporate ladder in a large bureaucratic system like the United Nations is just not possible. I am resigned to that! Why do I look up to *A* so much? Why do I say that *Z*'s generous act of giving the most sincere hug was a perfect example of why I needed, and continue to need, mentoring in my life? As much as I would like to praise them just for the heck of it, there is a point I want to make!

What is the value-added service of mentors? What do they do for us? As I thought more about my relationship with *A* and *Z*, I came across an article on FastCompany.com (https://www.fastcompany.com/3042664/the-five-types-of-mentors-you-need) that said there are five types of mentorship:

"THE COACH

There are times when you need someone to help you think through difficult problems. A good coach doesn't solve your problems for you. The coach listens to what you say, and asks you questions to help you dig through what might be causing those problems. Coaches can suggest strategies for solving problems you might not have considered, but in the end you are the one that has to implement them and (eventually) internalize those strategies to be used in the future.

THE STAR

Find people who have the career that you want. Spend time with them. Get to know how they operate, what they think about, how they prepare for big events.

THE CONNECTOR

It really is who you know in life that helps you move forward. In order to make sure that you build up your own list of contacts, find the people around you who know everyone.

THE LIBRARIAN

A good librarian knows how to find every book in the library. As you navigate your organization and the community around it, you need to know the resources that are available to help you along.

THE TEAMMATE

Some days you eat the bear. Some days the bear eats you. On those days where the bear got you, it's helpful to have someone who understands you and where you are in your career who can listen to what happened. Maybe you aren't looking for a solution or a motivational speech — just some validation that you had a tough day.

To be honest, I have never thought of *A* or *Z* in such classifying ways, but now that I have read the above article, I feel totally vindicated for having chosen them. They totally fit the bill on all five categories! I didn't choose them to play any of the specific roles above. I needed their help and their expertise, but I had never thought of what I was looking for in such clear-cut ways. As it turned out, I could not be luckier!

But why does anyone need a mentor? Does everyone need a mentor? Why did I need their mentoring in the first place? When I look back at some half century of my life, there are probably two things that have always been constants in my life. The first is that I have long believed in the "concept" of "success" in life. I put them in quotation marks because they are both very subjective terms and mean different things to different people. I am sure I did not know it back when I was a kid, but I think the idea of having to be successful was probably engrained in me from a very early age. That in itself is very strange because no one in my family had such inklings. There was no super ambitious person who could have inspired me, someone who would have played even a passive role model character in my life. So, where did it come from? I don't have a clue! And it was not just me knowing that I had higher aspirations. Just about everyone in my family talked about how I would "go places," without anyone having anything specific in mind.

And to achieve those high goals for myself, knowing that I lacked the skills and intellectual maturity at times, I knew that I needed help. I needed role models, and I was more than happy to not only accept them, but also to seek them. Let me explain this a bit more.

My first love in life was journalism. It is a profession that I think, from a philosophical standpoint, is the most honest and most impactful of the positions and careers I have had in life. Forget about how it is actually being practiced in many countries, including in my own country, the United States. I am talking about principles. I entered the media world at the age of nine as co-host of a five-day-a-week children's TV program. To this day, I remember how the audition went. Even at that early age, I had a busy life. I was on the chess team. I was on the gymnastics team. And, of course, I was going to school full time. I don't remember how I got to know about the advertisement for the television show, but I do remember my mother's reaction when I asked her to take me to the audition. Her response was something to the effect of, "Don't you have enough going on? Why do you want to add one more task? How will you manage?" But I insisted and she gave in. The day of the audition, some kids had already taken the audition and, I think, I was halfway in the queue. When my turn came, the organizers took me to a studio and told me to look at the camera and read from a script. By the time I finished, they were impressed enough to give me the job on the spot. The rest, as they say, is history. After three years as the TV co-host, I went to radio, then to newspapers and news agencies, then back to newspapers, with radio in between.

By the time I left journalism in 2005 at the age of forty-three, I had traveled to over three dozen countries and been in the thick of some major international news events, from the Iranian Revolution in 1979–80 and the Israeli invasion of Lebanon in 1982 to the Gulf wars and the 2003 invasion of Iraq. I have some truly gutsy and accomplished journalist friends, and I think they would agree that all good journalists are ambitious. They want to be successful. Success is engraved in our psyche, whether we think about it or not. Why else do we compete with each other to get the story first?

As with the UN, I had, and still have, role models in the world of journalism. That none of them is still a practicing and full-time journalist is simply a reflection of two things. First, we are all getting older, and second, journalism has changed so much that most of us have simply left the field. Regardless, my journalism experience once I had emigrated to the United States could not have progressed had I not met role models such as my former boss at the *Washington Post*, from whom I learned an immense amount, who mentored me and taught me lessons, who also gave me room to prove myself. Especially when talking about a practical field such as journalism, it is massively important to have role models and mentors who can teach you the ropes but to also watch you practice the trade and learn from it. There are probably half a dozen people in and out of the *Post* who played a large role in my development as a journalist to whom I am indebted.

Mentors should be credited with the good things that you get out of life. What life does not give you is not their fault. There is a lot to be said about the fact that I did not really "make it" in journalism the way I wanted to. I covered good stories, but I was never a full-time correspondent for any major national news organization. I worked for the *Washington Post* but was not given the chance to become one of its foreign correspondents. I covered the hostage crisis in Iran for The Associated Press but failed for years to get a full-time job with the news agency. I covered much of the 2003 Iraqi invasion for Radio Free Europe/Radio Liberty but could not get a staff job at their Prague, Czech Republic, headquarters, which is what I really wanted. And on and on and on. You get the picture! I know that there is little correlation between being a good journalist and being a full-time staff reporter for a major—or even not major—news organization, but that is the dream I had.

Back to the United Nations. I had my eyes fixed on the UN long before I left journalism. Why? For several reasons. In no particular order, first because of the lifestyle. I always had this idealistic notion that joining the UN would ensure mobility around the world every few years. That sounded exciting to me. After all, that was one of the reasons I loved the idea of being a foreign correspondent. As it turned out, that is not really the UN model, even though the organization always talks about mobility as a cornerstone of its human resources principles. It's a load of you know what. When you get a UN job, I learned, be prepared for one of the two things: stay where you are for years and years, or be prepared to quit after a while. In far too many cases, when you get a job in the UN system, you either sit on it for too many years because you are having a decent life in decent city, or you get a job in a not-so-desirable country and then get stuck for a *long* time, unable to find a job somewhere else because people in more desirable cities are not going anywhere and, therefore, there are no vacancies.

The second reason I was so keen to join the international organization was that I have always believed in the work of the United Nations. One must remember that when we talk about the UN, we are not just talking about fancily dressed men and women doing-whatever-they-do in that prime real estate in New York's East 42nd Street. Or in posh Geneva. The overwhelming majority of UN staff work for either numerous specialized agencies around the world or UN secretariat branches like the peacekeeping and political missions across the globe. While the diplomatic and political work that is done in New York and Geneva is tremendously important—and often controversial and mired in international politics—the work of the rest of the UN system is, arguably, much more important for people around the world.

A lot of times these agencies, most often wrongly but sometimes with some justification, also get caught in international politics. They get their work criticized unjustly. Just think of the criticisms about why humanitarian aid does not reach enough people or the right people in times of crises around the world. Or why the UN gives hope to refugees who flee their homelands only to land in countries that either don't want them or can't handle them. Or how some agencies end up inadvertently helping dictatorships, etc., etc.

So, yes, I have been eager to climb up the proverbial UN ladder for years, both out of professional commitment and for personal expediency. As of this writing, I think, realistically speaking, that dream is dead. At the age of fifty-seven, being white, male, and American, chances of success in the UN system for someone who lost whatever growth chances he had when power-hungry, back-stabbing, and disloyal bosses in my job in The Hague ended my career, are pretty nil.

But even with that, I could not have learned the lessons I did without the mentorship of *A* and *Z*. We, as human beings, normally do not think of mentorship as a daily dose of our life. The overwhelming majority of us don't wake up in the morning thinking "Whom can I mentor today?" or "I really need a mentor myself today. Whom can I choose?", but in fact, mentoring is much more widespread than we might think. And it is not limited to *nobodies* like me. Bill Gates had a mentor. So did Steve Jobs. Or even Elizabeth Taylor!

One of the better research papers on the topic I read—and I read many!—was published in the April 2008 issue of the *Journal of Vocational Behavior*. The findings in that paper, and others I read, solidified what I had suspected: we adopt or provide mentoring to decrease unwanted behavior and results and increase desired ones. (In my case, the latter!) Needless to say, there are many forms of formal and informal mentoring. The research paper focused on the three most common types: youth mentorship, academic mentorship, and work mentorship.

If I combine the "why" and "how" in seeking mentors, I should openly admit that I needed and wanted both youth and work mentorship because of who I was and have been. As I mentioned above, I was a rather ambitious person from a very young age who did not have that system of guidance from people who normally play such a role: my own parents, close family and relatives, or schoolteachers. When it came to being ambitious and wanting to "be someone" and achieve success in life, I was way ahead of the pack compared to anyone around me when I was a kid or a teenager. Many countries and educational systems have built-in mentorship programs for kids and teenagers before they enter the work environment, but I received a combined youth and professional mentorship for the first time when I was nineteen and had already fled Iran for Lebanon, where I ended up working for the American news agency United Press International.

In fact, the first two mentors I had—encompassing both youth and work mentorship roles—were people who have become my *de facto* guardians in the United States. I remember vividly and clearly my days—our days together—in Lebanon between 1981 and 1983. I am not sure and don't remember if I showed it or not, but I watched them and their behavior—how they interacted with each other, how they interacted with me, how they interacted with others. I was eager to learn. I knew I had a lot to learn, and I wanted to learn. There is no doubt in my mind that I was eagerly seeking mentorship.

Granted, I never had a normal childhood or teenage years, but looking back at my life and the years that I taught at various universities, I can attest that youth mentorship is probably the most important of the mentorship types. I have lost track of how many students I have had who, at one point or another during our time together, felt a sense of loss. Not knowing where they were going. Not knowing where they wanted to, or should, go. Not knowing how to get there, even if they knew what they wanted in life. How to gain and learn the skills that would help get them there. In that sense, I was lucky because I always knew what I wanted and, for the most part, had the skills to do the job. Whether I eventually succeeded or not, that was a different story, because there were other factors in the play. In return, I always tried to help my students as much as I could. I don't necessarily put those assistances in the mentorship column. Most of the time, it was just being their friend, talking, and passing on the experiences I had, but I hope it helped someone somewhere down the road!

Success is very close to the concept of dreams and ambition, and many people—myself included for a long time—associate the idea of accomplishing their dream with achieving success. But accomplishment and success are in fact rather distinct from each other. And that is another reason why mentorship is so important in my opinion. In that sense, a good mentor is almost like a psychiatrist, helping the "patient" or "mentee" not only understand the difference—and thus not be frustrated prematurely—but also help when he or she can with the accomplishment part. I, for one, have only learned that lesson in the past few years. To me, it goes back to the short-term hope versus long-term hope. Accomplishment, I would argue, is similar to short-term hope, for the most part. Success is a much more long-term track record of series and sequences of accomplishments.

I must admit that when I was in journalism, I was thinking of "success," but I really had "accomplishment" in mind on a day-to-day basis. Aside from the overall notion of wanting to be a recognized foreign correspondent, much of my focus was on doing a good job every day. As long as I was going from country to county and writing good, informative stories for the benefit of the public, I thought I was successful. There, too, my mentors were instrumental. They, whether the ones I have mentioned or many others from whom I have learned over the years, drilled into me the value of the principles of journalism, the value of the public service factor of the job, and the profession's societal impact.

Once in the UN, *A* and *Z*, were priceless in showing me the overall good that the international organization, and each of us in our particular jobs, were doing to make the world a better place, to give the societies in which we were working long-term assistance that would change their way of life for the better: how we contributed to providing better health services, how we protected the civilians from getting caught in senseless military and militia conflicts, how we helped girls get better education, how we helped change men's mindsets by showing them that violence against girls and women is wrong. Those were things you could count as day-to-day successes but also as long-term accomplishments.

Leaving journalism and entering the UN did not end the need for mentors. It reinforced it. When I was in journalism, the field was familiar to me. When I joined the UN, on the other hand, the "system" was totally new to me. I didn't know how the UN worked. More than any other time, I badly needed people like *A* and *Z*. They are still the perfect role models for me. My first job was, simply put, painful. I mean that in the literal, physical sense. The headquarters—New York—in its infinite wisdom, had sent us a new boss who was an absolute nightmare and drove everyone mad. Eventually, it got so bad that they quietly pushed her to retirement. That is when *A* and *Z* showed up in my life. *A* was a godsend. Not only because he helped me transfer to another position, but because I was beginning to learn—and am still learning—the ropes from him. I was learning from both of them everything from how to behave in the UN environment to what was a reasonable expectation and what was unreasonable. Mind you, reasonable and unreasonable in the UN world do not necessarily correspond to our common life definitions. The UN is a world in itself.

The more I got to know *A*, the more I admired him. He often tried to help me get jobs (and often did not succeed, which says something about the UN), but I don't admire him just because he tried to help me with jobs. He is my role model for who he is. He is genuinely kind and considerate. I have learned many lessons just watching how he works over the past years, mainly in being humble, showing humility, and putting the cause before the personal issues. I have tried to keep those lessons in mind in my own dealings with others.

As with *A, Z* showed me the value of trying to keep your calm in the UN system as much as possible. One of my worst experiences in the UN system was when a supervisor called me late at night on a Saturday. The week before had already been a tough week. She had given me a hard time about having done things that she had told me to do but then forgot that she had. I took the rap, because by then I had learned that to take it in and not have a confrontation was less painful—and it was the UN way of doing things, for the most part. The second the supervisor started talking when she called, I could tell she was drunk, or damn close to it. To be honest, as I write these lines, I don't remember the details of the conversation. I do remember her starting the call in a very prosecutorial and interrogatory tone. She was trying to put me on the defensive, and she was succeeding. Being inexperienced as I was in dealing with such situations, my defensive answers led to showing my anger. I could hear my voice rising. By then she was screaming. I had just gotten over a case of malaria and had not completely regained my physical health. I remember that somewhere in the middle of her screaming I started feeling deep pain in my stomach, as if someone had struck me with a sharp knife and was turning it around inside me for maximum impact. I could not take it anymore, and at some point simply hung up on her and started crying, both out of anger and the pain in my stomach.

Then, over the years, I remember the Zen-like atmosphere in *A*'s and *Z*'s offices every time I visited them and recall thinking to myself, "They certainly have lot of pressure on them, but none of it seems to be passed on to their staff. They all seem to be doing their own work." I've always tried to remember that when dealing with my own colleagues and staff. I am not saying I never made my staff nervous. I know I did. I remember when I was in The Hague, I had a young, female Lebanese colleague. I respected her a lot, and still do. She, too, had several qualities I could have used. In many ways, the section I was hired to run needed corrective measures, and that meant that I was putting pressure on the staff to make those changes. She took the brunt of my pressure and did so with grace and calm. She was reflecting the humility that I had seen in *A* and *Z*. I should have learned by then to possess them myself, but I had not. I was wondering how I could enforce the changes without being too pushy, let alone appearing as arrogant. The contrast between who I wanted to be, based on what I had learned from *A* and *Z*, and how my Lebanese colleague was reacting to my pressure has never been lost on me, and I often make a precise effort to re-evaluate my own behavior.

As of this writing, it is fair to say that I have failed in accomplishing what I had dreamed for myself, which was to rise up in ranks within the UN system to reach my own ambitions but also to be able to give back what I think I am capable of in my own capacity. As my long months of unemployment dragged on in 2016, one question remained on my mind and gained force.

Mentors

(By Jack Lennon)

Mentorship is a very important component of life, regardless of one's field of work. Learning from people who share interests and engage in the same type of activities, but are more senior in terms of experience, can propel one forward. This type of relationship differs from a friendship because there is a power differential, in most cases, but it can hold the same amount of value. This is especially true for those who are embarking upon competitive careers and aspirational life goals. Mentors do not always fall into one's lap, though, such that cold-calls or emails may be necessary to find a way into the network. It is this networking that can not only help locate mentors, but can help one develop his or her own name in a given field.

The concept of needing five types of mentors, even if the qualities can be found within a single individual, is a meaningful idea: 1) the coach, 2) the star, 3) the connector, 4) the librarian, and 5) the teammate (Markman 2015). Mentorship is defined in various ways, and this can be viewed as one of them. Mentorship is known to improve student efficacy and leadership ability (Lester et al., 2011) but should always be tailored to the individual's needs. Simply stated, the individual must be met where he or she is at. If one is relatively experienced, mentorship should start there, while if someone is new to the field, mentorship should start from the basics. The types of mentors noted above can all be helpful at any stage, so long as they are tailored, and the mentors are willing to take on this role. If one is fortunate enough to have people similar to *A* and *Z*, they should certainly take full advantage of all learning opportunities; learn and accept information without expecting payment or anything more. What one gains from these relationships will likely be much more beneficial than going about the process alone.

Mentors need not be those related to a professional realm; they can be life mentors who can assist in finding a path that suits one's interests and goals. This is important for all to consider, especially if professional mentorship does not seem to apply. For example, mentorship among adults living with spinal cord injuries reported increased physical activity, positive diet changes, as well as decreased stress, anxiety, and overall mental health (Shi et al., 2018). Similar studies have found similar improvements in quality of life (Hoffmann et al., 2019). There are always people who have been in similar positions and have found their ways to rewarding lifestyles.

Lastly, one should never undermine his or her abilities to serve as a mentor to others. This is a form of imposter syndrome, which occurs in countless fields. When a student earns a degree and begins to work with full autonomy, supervising others, it can feel unusual, to put it mildly. One may question why he or she is being given this opportunity—"What could I possibly offer? I'm an amateur." But the reality is that many of us feel this way initially, and we feel that way at several points in life; learning requires doing. Once one has developed a set of skills, those skills will continue to improve and be built upon, but the position one obtains is because he or she is capable of performing in that position. One's capabilities are often of much greater magnitude than initially perceived.

Should one feel substantial pressure and the feeling of being an imposter does not dissipate over time, ongoing mentorship can be used to discuss these thoughts. It can be useful to have discussions about feeling ill-equipped, and mentors will likely provide their own examples of feeling similarly—they were once in the same position. There is no need to limit oneself in the realm of helping others simply because it feels unusual or because skills do not match those of one's own mentors. Of course they don't, but they likely will. Seek consultation with your own mentors, and embrace the opportunity to pay it forward, should that be one's desire or calling.

References

Hoffmann, D. D., Sundby, J., Biering-Sørensen, F., & Kasch, H. (2019). Implementing volunteer peer mentoring as a supplement to professional efforts in primary rehabilitation of persons with spinal cord injury. *Spinal Cord, 57*(10), 881-889. https://doi.org/10.1038/s41393-019-0294-0

Lester, P. B., Hannah, S. T., Harms, P. D., Vogelgesang, G. R., & Avolio, B. J. (2011). Mentoring impact on leader efficacy development: A field experiment. *Academy of Management Learning & Education, 10*(3), 409-429.

Markman, A. (2015). The five types of mentors you need. Fast Company. Retrieved from https://www.fastcompany.com/90487967/were-just-doing-our-best-to-adapt-emma-straub-on-running-an-indie-bookstore-amid-coronavirus (accessed April 11, 2020).

Shi, Z., Rocchi, M., McBride, C. B., Shaw, R., & Shaw, S. (2018). Health outcomes of receiving peer mentorship for adults living with spinal cord injury: A qualitative meta-synthesis. *Exercise Psychology, 50*(1). Retrieved from https://www.scapps.org/jems/index.php/1/article/view/2001

But Are You Any Good?!

May 18, 1985, was a super day. It was a day that I was proud of myself. I was living in a small studio apartment up on Connecticut Avenue in northwest Washington, DC. I had woken up that morning around 6:00 a.m., as I had every morning that week, earlier than usual, to go downstairs and see if my copy of the *Washington Post* had arrived.

I did not really have to do that. I worked at the *Post*, and I could have easily waited a couple of hours more and read a free copy. But I was anxious. I opened the entrance door to the street and went outside. Even though that January had registered record-breaking cold in several parts of the country, including in Washington, that May morning was already a mild day, around 60 degrees Fahrenheit, about 15 degrees Centigrade.

My paper was there, wrapped in plastic and with my name on it. Instinctively, I jumped into the foreign news section. There it was, on page A15, the very top of the left side of the page, a story with the headline: "Split Apparent in Iran's Leadership Over Ways to End War Against Iraq". The cherry on the top: a box marking the story as "News Analysis". The byline: "Peyman Pejman,

Special to The Washington Post". To say that I was proud of myself would be an understatement. I had submitted the story probably a week earlier but didn't know when it would appear in the paper, so I had been waiting for it all week.

While it was not my first story in the *Post*, it was my fist analysis story, which, at least to me, carried a bigger significance. News analyses are usually done by mature journalists with many years of experience, and the stories are usually done from the field where the reporter can physically talk to various sources in one or more countries. I was a twenty-three-year-old "kid" at the time and was sitting at my Washington desk thousands of miles away from the Middle East. I was working full time and going to the university to get my bachelor's degree. I was working hard towards transitioning to being an American with high hopes and high dreams for a better and more successful journalism career.

As for the "Special to The Washington Post" designation, it was special not because of me but because I was *not* a *Post* reporter in the first place. I was what they used to call a "Copy Aide," someone who had administrative roles on the foreign desk. But my boss, a multiple Pulitzer-Prize-winning journalist with impeccable journalistic and intellectual streaks, had mentored me ever since I had started working at the *Post* the previous year and allowed me to write stories.

By the time I left the *Post* in 1987, I had published more than a dozen stories in the paper's foreign news pages; several of them had appeared on the front page of the section, and many were reprinted for worldwide distribution by the *International Herald Tribune*, which was co-owned by the *Washington Post* and The *New York Times*.

My shift at the *Post* started at 8:30 a.m. but for two weeks before I turned in my story, I had woken up at 5:00 and been at desk by 6:00 so I could spend a couple of hours working on the story, doing research, making overseas phones to places like Iran and Lebanon, and to write and rewrite the story until I was satisfied. I had to make sure that my *ad-hoc* writing would be done on my own time and not interfere with my official duties.

That day, I knew I was a good journalist, in great part because I had good mentors.

So, when I was writing the previous chapter about *A* and *Z*, I was very mindful that just wanting to be "great" and "successful" does not necessarily mean you deserve it, even if you work hard. And I am not saying that to be harsh on myself, although I am my own harshest critic.

While I had always dreamed of being a staff foreign correspondent, I never associated the fact that I did not rise up to that level with lack of skills. Sure, I needed to develop some skills, but I was willing to work for it if someone gave me a chance. I had the confidence, so did not equate the lack of materialization of my dreams with not having deserved them.

The UN was a different story. As I said before, I had never worked for the organization and was unsure of myself. To compensate for that, and to prove to myself as much as to others that I could do it, I worked really hard in my first two jobs. I delved right into the work and gave it my all. I did the same when I worked for a tribunal in The Hague. In fact, The Hague job was even more daunting for at least two reasons. First, it was the highest-ranking position I had held in the UN, and I needed to prove that I was up to the task, in part because it involved a higher level of management skills as well as programmatic knowledge. Second, tribunals and international courts are truly beasts of a different nature. They are divided into at least three sections (organs, as they call them) – the Registry, which runs the administration; Prosecution; Chambers, which includes the judges; and sometimes the Defense. Each is headed by someone appointed directly by the UN secretary-general (at the recommendation of some other office or person), and to say that they usually have enough ego to consider themselves gods on earth would not be too much of an exaggeration. (The prosecutor in that tribunal was the only down-to-earth and truly decent human being of all the senior management.) To do a good job in communications at tribunals is a herculean task just because of the set-up alone, among other reasons. I knew that, and I was doing my best not only to navigate the system but also to push the organization to where I thought it should go from the communications perspective. Did I learn all the right lessons? Would I say I was successful in it? I clearly learned a lot, but I also made mistakes. Did I know enough and had learned enough to deserve the job? Absolutely.

People like *A* and *Z* and my journalism mentors reach high places because they work hard, because they are good at what they do, and yes, because someone somewhere down the road probably gave them a break and opened some doors for them. In the twelve months that I was unemployed, and particularly in the last four or five months of it, I often thought about the issue of "deserving success" in my life in general and in the UN in particular. Was I thinking about suicide because I had not reached professional zenith? The answer is a resounding no, but I have learned a few things about myself and about the relationship between ambition and the level of frustration that leads to the thoughts of suicide.

In the article I cited before from the *PsychCentral* website, there was also this:

"Our depression is a comparison of our current reality to a fantasy that we are addicted to. If that fantasy is extremely unreasonable and unobtainable, thoughts of suicide can emerge. And the longer the fantasy is held onto and the more we are addicted to it, the more the depression can linger, and the more the thought of suicide can become the only way out . . . So any time we have an expectation that is delusional or extremely unrealistic, or is not aligned with our true, highest values, depression can ensue and suicide can become a persistent thought. Many have had moments where they have contemplated and considered it."

In simple terms, I found myself asking, "Kid, do you deserve the life and the lifestyle you want, and for which you've been trying hard?" For me, in that stage of my life, this was a very existential question. It was not *pro forma.* It was not hypothetical. I can assure you that I have given it massive amount of thinking. Were my expectations unrealistic? Was I delusional? Was I aspiring to something that was clearly out of my reach? Overall, I would say no, I don't think I was overreaching.

There is another topic that has direct relevance to the role of mentors and how they can clarify things for the mentees. I have spent a lot of time researching whether overly ambitious people are inherently more depressed. In other words, is it just part of life that because you have high ambitions, that you suffer more probably because you fall more often than "normal" people? This is a slippery-slope argument for several reasons. First because, as I mentioned above, there are a zillion reasons why one might be frustrated, or even suffer from longer-term depression, but they are not necessarily chronic depression. Just because you go through bouts of depression even for a couple of years for specific reasons related to job or whatever, it does not mean you are a chronically depressed person. So, you can have high ambitions in life, fall a few times here and there and be super-frustrated or depressed because of it, but that does not make you naturally and automatically prone to depression. The other reason that tying high ambitions with depression is a slippery slope is that extreme depression, if not treated early, can easily turn into mental illness. A wide host of famous artists—Lady Gaga, Selena Gomez, etc.—have admitted that once they achieved the fame they so desired, they then had to deal with severe depression and think of mental health issues.

Now, obviously, I am no Lady Gaga and will never be, but one does not have to be Lady Gaga to wonder whether the price of achieved or not achieved ambition is depression, and whether that can lead to worse things such as wanting to commit suicide. Again, do I believe my suicidal thoughts had anything to do with my unmaterialized ambitions? I would say on the surface of it, no. Could it be that on some subconscious level I was using my financial difficulties as another manifestation of my long-suppressed angst for not having achieved my dreams, and thus pushing myself towards suicide? Maybe.

Back to the question of whether I deserve to have my dreams come true. One of the things I have learned in the past decade or so in my life is when to quit the proverbial poker game. In other words, learn when I wanted something that was not going to happen and stop wanting it! So, for the next few paragraphs, I am going to assume that the answer is "No," that I don't deserve the life I want and give you examples of when I might have been overreaching, but also when I thought it was feasible, given help and the kind of mentoring I mentioned in the previous chapter.

The two examples I am going to mention illustrate a time when I was way out of my depth and another time when success was feasible but required a combination of luck, help, and hard work. Both could have used more mentoring.

The first example moves me back to the summer of 1996 when I moved back to Washington, DC, after five and a half years of successful and somewhat lucrative journalism freelancing and teaching in Cairo, Egypt. I loved living in Egypt, and hard as the freelancing business was, I had gotten the hang of it and was living a fun life, working hard, partying, and having friends in Egypt's High Society. But I felt that I had been in Egypt too long and needed to make a move to take my life and my career to the next level. Within a couple of years after my return to Washington, I had left journalism, was getting my master's degree in Information Technology, working as a technical writer for IT companies, and had decided to open my own IT company. I thought journalism had changed so much that I could not prosper in it any longer the way I wanted to—and I wanted to make more money. It was perhaps the first time in my life that I was putting making money at the forefront of the vision for my future. The American dream, the desire for material success, was finally catching up with me. And because I was then about forty, the pressure was double and triple. I felt I had to make up for the lost time, and do it fast.

The idea I had for my IT company was good then, and it is still good: Provide an online business-to-business platform that would introduce businesses in the Middle East to their counterparts in Europe and the United States and facilitate their trade, including sales transactions. But while the idea was good, the set up was not. I did not have previous business experience, so I was not doing a good job of getting the project off the ground. It was a technology and software-based project, so it needed a team. I did not have reliable partners. I tried to interest a few people so we could organize a board, but in reality, their heart was not in it, or they did not buy the idea and just did not have the heart to tell me, so they just played along. I spent a bunch of my own money, raised about $30,000 as a loan from someone, and ended up declaring personal bankruptcy (but paid off the $30,000 from my savings in later years). So, that was my first lesson outside journalism, shooting high and falling hard. And it was my fault. I did not do it right and learned many lessons from it.

The second time I questioned whether I had what it takes to be who I want to be was shortly after I joined the United Nations. Having waited for years to join the UN, within a short few months I was begging people to get me out of my first assignment. Granted, as I mentioned before, the boss was the craziest person anyone had seen in a while, but that did not mask the fact that I was failing in coping with a bad situation when many of my other colleagues who had been in the system much longer and had developed a thicker skin were faring better. I remember the message I received in a meeting I had with someone in the senior management before I finally received a lateral transfer and left for another assignment: "You know, if you want to leave, we won't stop you, but you should know that the peacekeeping life is not for everyone." I remember thinking at the time, "You are supporting this maniac (my boss) who is making everyone's life miserable, and you are calling me a wimp for wanting to move on?" But he did have a point!

Ten months into my second twelve-month contract, I decided to quit my job. To be sure, there were a series of reasons why I did so. The peacekeeping life was hard, but the hardship was not one of the reasons I quit. Everyone knew most of these peacekeeping missions were a hard life. Often—as was the case with my second job— people were living in tiny FEMA-style emergency containers with no private bathroom or shower. Showers were communal, and bathrooms were often so filthy that you would throw up before you were done. But even today, with the hindsight of many years of retroactive thinking, I still think I made the right decision to quit my job, even if that meant I was throwing in the towel and potentially giving up on the dream of working for the United Nations. In wanting so badly to work for the organization, I had not considered many factors. I had jumped into a situation about which I did not know as much as I should have. Just like my business experience, I had let my dream of doing something, my ambition, get the better part of me, but I ultimately failed because of my lack of adequate knowledge of what it takes to make success out of a complicated situation.

So, am I good enough to get what I want? Well, in the first instance, I clearly did not deserve it. The learning curve was too high. I did not have the basics covered. Much of the project's success depended on many other people, people I had not even identified or mobilized into a team. But the ambition, wanting to do good and rise up in the UN system was, and still is, doable. Help? Absolutely. Over my head? Definitely not.

The question of whether I am good enough to deserve my high dreams has brought me face to face with another reality. To repeat a poor metaphor, there is more than one way to skin a cat. There is more than one way to achieve your dream. I mentioned that my over-the-top fascination with wanting to work with the UN has to do with three things: 1)The work itself—helping people; 2)Going higher on the professional ladder, learning new skills and doing a better job; 3)Making decent money and making sure I have a good retirement. Well, not everybody works for the UN, and millions and millions of people get to satisfy all three of those desires. So, why not try another door, try another field? I don't know if I am the only one, or if it is even a trait that ambitious people become so fixated on one thing that they don't consider other options—sort of the tunnel-vision syndrome. But in my case, there actually is a field—other than journalism, which unfortunately does not pay enough to satisfy my last requirement, and the UN, in which I seem to have failed—that I can and have been trying. Teaching just might prove to be my salvation.

I got into teaching quite accidentally back in early 90s. I was working as a journalist in Egypt, and I knew the then chairman of the journalism department at the American University in Cairo—a very respected university in the Middle East—through social channels. One day, out of the blue, he asked me if I wanted to fill in for a teacher who had suddenly taken leave, and the university needed to find someone quickly to teach her course. I said yes. At first, it was a struggle. I found out very quickly that being a journalist is very different from teaching journalism. Teaching is a profession in and of itself. Being a practitioner and knowing the skills does not necessarily make you a good teacher, although it certainly is a prerequisite and goes a long way in making sure students respect you.

Over the years, I have taught a number of times and treasure the responsibility and enjoy the work. I like working with students, to tell them what I know, and perhaps influence a tiny minority. For a whole host of reasons, most of the students I have dealt with are not interested in journalism. Most are interested in public relations and communications. But I also like teaching for the same reasons that I have needed people like *A* and *Z*. That is, I like the idea that I can help some young souls benefit from some of the experiences I have gained in life. You might have noticed I did not use the word "mentoring." For me, the word is a heavy one and carries a lot of weight, and I simply do not want to allow myself to be put on the level of people like my own mentors. So, I am quite happy with phrases like "share experiences," "tell them about my experiences," "talk about what I have gone through and what I have learned from them." And my eight years of teaching has shown that I have had some success and influenced some students.

Ironically, one of the ways that I measure my own success is how many of my former and current students are also my friends. I did not tell any of my former student friends when I was going through difficult times. But I know that I will be there for any of my friends, should they be in trouble, and give them a meaningful hug the way *Z* did or give them advice the way *A* has given me. That makes me okay with staying in teaching, conveying knowledge and information, making friends, and lending a hand if needed some day. Exactly because of my own life experience, I totally reject the idea that teachers are there to teach and not become friends with students. Respect boundaries inside the class, absolutely. But unless they trust you and feel comfortable with you, they won't accept you as a lifelong mentor. They would need to get to know you, and know you well, first, and for that, the relationship has to expand beyond the classroom. I know there are many professional and career academics who disagree with me on this, but I am firmly sticking to my guns on this point.

Perhaps if one is in a formal mentoring program, then there might not be a need for bonding or friendship, but in my case, I have benefitted from both. What I mean is that when I was in journalism, the bosses and colleagues who helped me grow and taught me many things at the *Washington Post* were not my friends. To this day, while I still have maintained my relationship with several of them, it is more of a relationship with people I respect. Others were friends and mentored me because they were my friends.

It might sound kind of obvious to psychiatrists or psychoanalysts but the time that I have questioned most whether I am good enough was the many months that I was looking for a new job, when I was unemployed in 2016. With a few exceptions here and there, during those very, very long months, I was applying to between five and ten jobs a day, usually seven days a week. That means between January and end of 2016, I must have applied to over two thousand jobs. I did not limit myself to applying for UN jobs. In fact, right from the start, I cast the net very wide. I applied for UN positions, for communications positions with non-governmental organizations, non-profits, universities (as I have mentioned, I had taught so had academic background), private sector media and communications jobs, and even a few journalism jobs.

But it would be foolish not to recognize my own shortcomings. As I think I have said before, I jumped too many branches, didn't stay in career tracks long enough to be able to make an impact or deserve it, with the exception of journalism. (In addition to academia, I had tried to get into the US Foreign Service. So, with journalism, UN, and academia, I had tried four different career paths!) This may be a small example, but it is an evidence in the question "Are you good enough?" During all those months that I sent out so many CVs, I probably didn't tailor-make my CVs and cover letters as much as I should have. Instead of mass-mailing CVs, maybe I should have concentrated more on a few of the best job vacancies. Maybe I should have worked harder on the two or three interviews that I actually did get but messed up.

But that takes me back to the topic of the chapter, mentoring, and the situation that COVID-19 has created for many millions of people. I have mentioned that one reason I made *A* and *Z* the centerpiece of my thinking about my own career path is that they stuck to a field of their interest through thick and thin. I did not. But if you think about it, if I were one of the many millions of people who have lost their job because of the current virus crisis, I would probably be in a better position to find something—even temporarily—than many of the people who have had one career track in their life. In the process of making a mess out of my own life, I also have learned different skills well enough to qualify for different jobs.

That is another aspect to the "Are you good enough" argument, and that is the changing nature of employment markets and factors that are beyond our own control. While I have praised the UN, I should also be honest and criticize its hiring practices, and this goes for nearly all specialized agencies as well as the Secretariat. There is no doubt that I—and virtually every other person I know whether in or out of the system—is frustrated with the international body's hiring practices. The UN as a whole is known for having one of the least transparent hiring systems. While I don't have provable statistics, I would venture to guess that half of the UN jobs are already decided by the time vacancy notices are put out. Call it corruption or whatever you want. And when it is not decided, it is *very* common for the hiring process to take six, nine, or twelve months from the time it is advertised. I mention that for those of us who blame ourselves for not being able to get the jobs we feel we deserve and don't; not everything is within our control to begin with.

The employers who fired their employees when the coronavirus pandemic started and will at some point start to rehire again, will they give preference to the employees they had, or will they opt for hiring less-experienced, younger people who will bring in less experience but will also be happy with lower salaries? Where would that put people like me?

But Are You Any Good?!

(By Jack Lennon)

Based on what we know about clinical depression—the negative mood and thoughts (self-talk)—when it is placed in the context of achievements, it is understandable to imagine questioning "are you any good?" This is a very difficult question, though one could argue that being good enough is only a fraction of what is necessary for certain accomplishments. Let's not forget the need for the random luck involved in life. One may have put in the work but is not having the best of luck. There are likely situations in which it is very difficult to accomplish certain goals based on factors beyond our control. Two clear examples seem apropos, each of which describe very concrete but external forces working against the achievement. For example, if one is thirty-two years of age, it is currently impossible to be the president of the United States; one must be at least thirty-five years of age. Sure, an individual can wait another three years, but the intention of this example is to provide a very clear example of limiting factors. The next example is the person who wishes to be an Olympic sprinter. This not only requires a lot of hard work and dedication in terms of training, but the reality is that this type of ability is based overwhelmingly in the genetics of fast-twitch muscle fibers. Not everyone can be a successful Olympic sprinter—the 100-meter, for example. These types of thought experiments, while simple and obvious, shed light on legitimate achievements that are unlikely. Most others that are rooted in other qualities are well within anyone's reach.

As one can likely tell at this point, whether or not one is *any good* depends almost entirely on how one thinks. One cannot think himself or herself into being older, but outlook matters. If the thought is not "I am good enough", it is possible that one's determination and drive will not be as ideal as necessary; it is difficult to wake up every day working toward something we do not deserve or we are not good enough to achieve. This can certainly be improved upon through mentors, which is where *A* and *Z* came into play. People who are in the field of choice can be honest and, if necessary, teach the necessary skills. When one is succeeding in a given field, it is far less likely for one to question his or her *goodness* or fit with the profession. Why question what's working well? It is when we face issues that we begin to reflect on why issues are arising, often turning fault inward and possibly outward. These are the loci of control—internal and external—both of which are common in depression as well as simple disappointment.

The referenced *PsychCentral* quote is comprised of some meaningful components but also uses suicide in such a way that it should be clarified. Suicide is often seen as a way out—an escape—from an otherwise intolerable situation or a life not lived according to our plans. But depression and suicide, while associated with one another, are many giant steps apart. It is also true, in my opinion, that people often live their lives not in the present but in some future moment. We are plagued by this forward-looking mindset that prohibits us from living in the current moment because we are too concerned with what we deserve at some future time. We are often just barely grasping the banister—waiting for X to occur or Y to happen, only to be met with another moment at which we start waiting for the next ideal moment. This is difficult to avoid when one is highly determined and motivated. It is understandable, though, given what we have discussed regarding setting goals and taking small steps toward future desires. How does one live in the present if one must also think about the future in the present moment? The simple answer is that it is easier said than done. But it is possible. Count every accomplishment.

Make goals so small and seemingly minor that they can be achieved on a daily or weekly basis. Count and celebrate those accomplishments, even if one is not yet sitting in his or her ideal position. One can move toward a future moment while appreciating and respecting the present moment. It is my opinion, but also a clinical phenomenon, that living in a moment that has not yet been granted can have negative impacts on one's mindset. Mindset could very well be negatively impacted if one is accomplishing nothing. Realize that the tasks of every single day are accomplishments, even if they are not overwhelmingly satisfying to those of us who are working toward a major dream.

This is also another moment for growth, for reflection. I would venture to say that most goals are not delusional. If one is truly questioning this, speak to someone in the field because these people know what it takes. Is a particular goal unrealistic? With such a large number of variables at play in life, it is difficult to determine what is realistic and what is not. Some barriers are set up to prevent people from accomplishing goals, while others find their ways around these barriers. Depression is certainly a difficult term to play with in this context, as it is both a general term to describe a state of emotion as well as a clinical diagnosis, which are very different. Falling short on a goal and feeling sad or disappointed is normative and expected; it is also expected that one should bounce back from these negative states. Depression is the inability to bounce back from these events. This highlighted comment has yet to be fully realized in studies; gaps between plans and attainment are not generally associated with depression. However, other characteristics can be—deeply insightful people who see the world for what it is are prone to feel sadness and depression. This sometimes comes with being a Type A personality, but in other cases, Type A personalities are tuned out of emotions. But again, do not forget that these are vague terms, and the qualities within these terms are more important.

Highly ambitious people are more likely to fail than those who take less risks—this is just basic common sense. Taking risks increases the likelihood of being rejected. As cliché as it may sound, rejections and failures do serve to teach lessons. Not all of them do; some are inappropriate and random. The vast majority of rejections, though, may suggest to us that something needs to change, whether they are small or large changes. Mentors can be supportive in these times, as they can not only share stories about their own inevitable failures, which is an experience that will travel throughout all of one's professional career, but mentors can also guide one in the right direction to reduce the likelihood of similar failures in the future. This will also serve to prevent one from feeling incompetent or ill-equipped to serve as a mentor himself or herself. This will serve to prevent one from feeling alone, delusional, or realistic in his or her endeavors. It is important to learn from mistakes, whether one can do that alone or through personal stories of others. The ultimate reality is that the philosophical question is this: *why wouldn't you deserve it?*

Pain

We must all suffer one of two things: the pain of discipline or the pain of regret or disappointment

Jim Rohn, American motivational speaker

Your pain is the breaking of the shell that encloses your understanding

Khalil Gibran

Sunday, November 6, 2016, was one of those bad days. I had not had a day like that in a few weeks. I had woken up thinking I was on a positive roll. The previous two days, I had maintained a decent balance between looking for a job, spending some time on freelance work—which made me feel useful and productive—and even exercised, spending time on the treadmill machine I had purchased the previous year, and doing as many sit-ups and push-ups as I could. So, I woke up that morning feeling okay. My health had been regressing the previous week or so, but I was mentally fit to fight it. But then something happened. What? I didn't know! I never knew those days, to be honest. Many months of unemployment and financial pressure, coupled with still-raw nerves over a difficult job before I became unemployed and poor health, had in some ways taken my life out of my control. I was fine one minute, and then, bang, I would lose control. It was even hard to say what the trigger was. Sometimes, it was just nothing. Sometimes, it was just an old memory or the thought of an old friend. Sometimes it was just a silly TV episode. And the tears would run down my face and wash it many times over. I would have problems breathing, my chest would start aching, and the pain deep inside my stomach would become so intense that it would exacerbate my crying, which by that point was likely an incessant sobbing. It was a vicious cycle of shedding tears, my chest aching, feeling like I was suffocating deep inside, and all I could do was to hold my head between my hands, lean on a table or a chair or a desk, and simply say to no one in particular, "Please, help me. Please, end this soon. Please, help me. Please, end this soon. I cannot do this much longer. Please, just help!" Sometimes, it took hours just to get over the physical pain and ensuing psychological instability before I could feel "normal" and continue my day.

Most times in the previous nine months, there might have been one episode like that in a given day, but that day once was not enough. I was fine for an hour or two, then it would start again. And again. And again.

That brings me to the question of pain itself. Why do we suffer pain? Why do we have to? Is there a correlation between the level of pain we are in and what we have or have not done in our past? Is pain only a physical phenomenon? Is there a way to measure how much more potent pain becomes when the physical and psychological get mixed up? Do we suffer pain as a form of guilt restitution? If so, is there a "price" on the restitution? Who would be the collector? Because, I tell you, I offered so many times in quiet and loud conversations with someone high above that I was happy to pay! Just tell me to whom and how much! I said so many times that I was happy and eager to pay for my past sins and mistakes. I know I have made mistakes, and I want to be a better person in life, so one of the things I have become rather conscious about in the past few years is to actually *be* a better person. I am not going to go through what I am doing and what I have done. That is between me and my conscience! I have even given this a lot of thought: could it be that I was being inflicted continuous pain by having my luck locked because my past guilts are so big? Is that why the restitution has taken this long, or might even continue much longer? It is hard to say, because I didn't know what exactly I was being punished for.

But, more importantly, I don't know what the punishment scale is! Is the punishment for having done Guilt *A*, the refusal on *B* number of job applications? Is the punishment for Guilt *C* incessant crying for *D* number of hours? If I mistreated someone, somewhere, sometime in the past, is that worth *F* number of hours of holding your stomach, bending on your knees, and wondering if you'd get up again? I don't know, but that's certainly something I have thought about a lot and will likely continue to do so.

And you might ask, "Why are you even equating pain with guilt?" Honestly, I am writing this chapter as a direct follow-up to the previous chapter, that I could not understand why I could not find a job and faced losing all my financial assets to the point of having to commit suicide. I could not accept any longer that not only was I not good enough for any UN job, but I was also not good enough for *any* other job. That no one would hire me to go back to journalism. That no one was giving me editing jobs. That no company or non-governmental organization thought I could help them with their communications tasks. That no university would hire me, even for a part-time job. I mean, what the hell? How was it possible that all of a sudden I had become totally unqualified for *every job*? In my own feeble mind, in that feeble physical, psychological, and vulnerable financial situation, the only thing I could think of was that I was being punished for something, even if it was for not believing in God and religions in the first place. The only way I could make sense out of the killing pain was to associate it with past mistakes, errors, sins, and guilts!

I chose the quotes at the beginning of this chapter on purpose and for a reason. Dictionaries would tell us that there are different types of pain, with the physical and mental being the most common ones. What no dictionary definition or article I have seen has done is to help me measure pain, or for that matter tell me when to recognize the start of some of the more subtle types of pain. And what is a real pain and what is a pain-like inconvenience. Is the first time you cry over a bad break-up or fight with a boyfriend or girlfriend a real pain or just a temporary inconvenience? I don't know the answer. In fact, I think no one should claim that he or she knows the answer because, to me, pain is a very personal thing. It is as unmeasurable as it is unique to each individual. And I say that because of the first quote above. I chose it because Jim Rohn, who was an American author and motivational speaker, seems to say that pain is a necessity in life. That he says "we must all suffer" some kind of pain implies that he equates pain with some rite of passage. In fact, I am pretty sure he meant that because of the second half of the above quote, that we must either suffer the pain of becoming or remaining disciplined in life, or suffer the pain of failing to do so. One way or another, he seemed to say that we are doomed!

The common assumption in many psychological and sociological circles is that if you are disciplined in life, you are naturally wired to want to be a high achiever, that you are destined to set your sights high, work harder, be more successful, and therefore be happier in life. After all, is that not how rich people have become who they are? Or top-notch politicians, or sportsmen and women, etc.? At least that's how I thought it would be in my life.

There is even literature linking ambition with living longer. A 2008 article in the British newspaper *The Observer* quoted a study published in *Health Psychology* as saying, "People who are industrious, disciplined and ambitious, live up to four years longer than those with more impulsive personalities . . . Conscientious types, often seen as boring, actually have the right personality to ensure that they live to a ripe old age." The research by renowned professor Howard Friedman of the University of California-Riverside found that order and achievement are two of the strongest indicators for living longer.

But it is not as carved in stone as one might think. In fact, there is also a lot of contrarian literature disputing that ambition and success equal happiness. One of the best-known scientific researches on the subject was the work of Timothy Judge, a professor of management at the University of Notre Dame's Mendoza College of Business. Judge, who studied 717 ambitious people, told *Fortune* magazine: "We discovered that ambition has, at most, only a very slight positive effect on life satisfaction, and actually a slightly negative impact on longevity." He added, "So, yes, ambitious people do achieve more successful careers, but that doesn't seem to translate into happier or healthier lives." He went on to say: "Occasionally, one encounters a concept that is pervasive yet poorly understood. Arguably, such is the case with ambition . . . Ambition has been discussed by numerous philosophers, with those seeing it as virtuous apparently outnumbered by those perceiving it as vicious."

What I found very interesting is the different interpretations of ambition based on who is studying it. As Judge said in his study, "In the case of ambition, understanding of the concept remains elusive . . . Psychologists have generally treated ambition as a trait, whereas sociologists have instead considered explicit educational or occupational objectives as a product of parental, social, or socioeconomic environment. We are aware of no studies that consider both personality-based and environmental sources of ambition. Nor are we aware—beyond those notable few who view ambition as a facet of conscientiousness or extraversion—of any studies that have sought to integrate ambition with the most influential typology in personality psychology."

And this was the kicker: "On the consequences of ambition, beyond the sociological aspirations literature noted previously, very few studies have linked ambition to career success, and we are aware of none that have linked it to intrinsic and extrinsic career success."

Apparently, even President Obama had something to say about the subject, saying ambition to achieve extrinsic success represents "a poverty of ambition . . . the elevation of appearance over substance, celebrity over character, short-term gain over lasting achievement." I think what the former president was saying is that there is a big difference between deep, meaningful, long-term achievement and short-term gain.

So, what does that all say about me? Considering that the literature seems to be far from conclusive on several issues, I think I will stick to my own ideas and beliefs on this for now! First off, I never did, and still do not, think about the relationship between ambition and longevity in life. I have had enough fun in life, had so many good and worldly experiences in so many countries around the world, that, frankly, I could not care less if I lived a few years longer or fewer. On happiness, it depends on who defines happiness. Again, terms such as "happiness," "success," or "pain" are so personal that I believe it should be left to each individual to set the yardsticks for himself or herself. For me, happiness is tied to the long-term success, which in turn translates to financial comfort. I don't want to become rich. Okay, if I win the lottery or one of my books becomes massively successful and I make lots of money from it, I won't complain, but making money in and of itself is not, and has never been, a measure of happiness for me.

Having worked since the age of nine and, as of this writing, not having secured a comfortable retirement scheme for myself, and not willing to downsize or lower my dreams by, say, selling my house in France and going to live in my condo in the States, financial comfort is everything to me— or at least figuring out a way that will get me there by the time I reach retirement age. I am not going to receive any inheritance money from anyone. I am single. The idea of being in my seventies and eighties and having no reliable retirement system very literally scares me to death and has been the source of much consternation for me in the past decade or so, and put a lot psychological pressure on me. Professional advancement and the sense of satisfaction in myself at achieving the best have been the source of my ambition and the measure of my happiness. But on that front, I am more or less okay, despite my failure in regard to the UN. I have done other things that I can be happy with, even though I recognize my mistakes and wish I could take them back.

So, finally, what do all these say about pain? I need to be conscientious enough to differentiate between anxiety and pain. Surely, we all go through different levels of anxiety in our lives. I suppose that is not only healthy but also necessary.

The experience of 2016 was profound. I had never gone through such an experience in my life. It tested me from every angle: moral, physical, psychological, professional, and, of course, financial. Honestly, I don't know if I can go through and survive such an experience if there is ever a second time. I certainly don't want it for myself, and I would never wish it on anyone else. I said not long ago that I have never wanted to be rich or super rich, but if anything changes dramatically in my life and I do make lots of money, helping people in this area would be a big priority of mine. I am not sure how exactly I would help. I don't have a specific project in mind as I write these lines, but I will look for ideas and projects to help people who fall down as deep as I did. Also, it does not have to be a big project. Helping people with even small amounts so it would change something, some temporary problem in their daily lives, is important. For me, even helping engineer such a small change would go back to letting someone have short-term hope about something for which they can be happy and thus call it a successful day. That's a promise I have made to myself, and that is part of the promise I made to myself to be a better person in life.

We all measure pain differently, and I don't have a problem with life testing us and our limit, but life, fate, gods, or whoever should not have the right to push us to point of breaking us.

Pain

(By Jack Lennon)

Pain is not *only* a physical phenomenon. Depression is a form of pain. But beyond that, all types of pain are subjectively experienced because of the brain. There is nothing fake about pain because the brain produces it. There are types of pain, even physical pain, that are unrelated to physical damage, which may be the question many ask. Depression, as merely one example, can come with aches and pains in various areas. The symptoms of depression are dependent on the individual and cultural norms. Those who come from cultures and environments that do not verbally express feelings are more likely to experience somatic complaints (complaints about physical pain). This is not because the pain is made up or not real, but because the depressive feelings have been translated or converted into physical symptoms. This happens in anxiety regularly. One can experience shakiness, sweating, agitation that requires pacing, headache, or lightheadedness. The anxiety is still a product of brain function. Where it ultimately ends up and how it is expressed does not change what it is.

We live in a social environment that stigmatizes mental health conditions for reasons that are not based in science. What one should be aware of, though, is that we know a great deal about depression and how it presents in the brain. The verdict is out that depression is a result of brain dysfunction—dysfunction that can be altered with various types of treatment. Those who believe that we still live in the 1950s, during which we also completely misunderstood dementia as people losing their minds, simply do not understand how far we have come. Never allow someone to claim that pain must come from a specific type of event. Much like a tumor, which is a noticeable, physical object, the same amount of damage can be caused through other brain issues that are related to its complex circuitry.

For example, guilt and shame are certainly types of pain that one may experience—they are not enjoyable states of being. The questions asked in the preceding chapter are important, philosophical questions: 1) how does one measure pain, 2) how does one recognize subtle forms of pain, and 3) what is the difference between real pain and a pain-like inconvenience?

1) Many of us will be familiar with the numerical rating scale for pain. Reporting a one is "no pain at all," while ten is considered "the worst pain

imaginable," two extreme poles. When it comes to psychical pain or pain due to mental health concerns, it may be more difficult to use this numerical system. We could certainly compare previous states and determine the best fit for the current state. Ultimately, much of these questions comes down to validating our own pain and describing the pain based on how we perceive it, not how we believe others will perceive it.

2) The hope is that one may be better suited to recognize more subtle forms of pain, as well as forthcoming pain, through the reading of these chapters. When one can validate pain in all its forms, as well as one's potential bases for the pain, one can use his or her knowledge to understand what may be a more nuanced form, a sign of more significant pain or concern. One cannot recognize that which has not yet occurred but can certainly reflect upon what is known. We each know ourselves better than anyone else; we know what feelings are typical for us, which are atypical for us, and how we define depression and suicide risk. Reflection is key here, and while there may not be perfect answers to every question, there are meaningful answers nonetheless.

3) This particular question is one that needs to be unpacked, so let us restate it here: *What is the difference between real pain and a pain-like*

inconvenience? The word *difference* already implies that the following states are assumed to be different, which may be untrue depending on what we are discussing. When it comes to *real pain* and a *pain-like inconvenience*, it is understandable that these two phenomena would be dichotomized, placing them on two separate poles along a continuum of pain. If we take this route, we can place a pain-like inconvenience at one on the pain scale; we can place real pain at a ten on that same scale. The fallacy here is that some of these states are valid forms of pain and others are not, when in fact they are all valid. When we experience pain, that very statement should suggest to us that we are experiencing pain. It need not be compared to the pain of others.

A common logical flaw is assigning value judgments to our painful experiences. "He or she experienced *X* and my experience right now is not nearly as bad as that." This simply is not true, because we are all different and, based on our experiences, we will invariably experience pain differently. It is accurate that a bad break-up or the death of a close relative or friend is different than depression—it is expected grief. In fact, we cannot diagnose MDD in the context of grief unless it extends beyond what is expected to be commensurate with the experiences of a specific individual in his or her context. Again, we are expecting that one should be able to bounce back from understandable sadness and depression. If it continues and one cannot bounce back, this is when we may be dealing with more than grief.

In all cases, when one believes that he or she is experiencing pain, it *is* pain, and no one should say otherwise. Pain comes in various forms, and they are all valid. We must recognize this, otherwise we may fall into a hole of feeling that we do not have the human right to experience all that life offers. Whether or not "we must all suffer" is a philosophical question that may harbor truth, depending on how one views the statement. Suffering can make some stronger; it may break down others in an unhealthy manner. Is suffering required to grow and learn? Maybe. Maybe not. It is not necessarily true that this world ought to make people suffer; one can potentially imagine an ideal world in which there is no suffering. Whether or not people would mature in the same ways or appreciate what they have in the same manners is a question that will likely remain unanswered, because the world in which we live is less than ideal. One can believe whatever he or she would like and will never be proven wrong, because they are both equally likely.

Before the next statements are made, it is important to understand how research studies in psychology, or any field, proceed with measuring variables. For a variable that has many definitions across individuals, such as happiness, studies must operationally define it; they must provide a definition that is being used in the study. Without a definition that makes the term operational, we do not know what is being measured. The same would apply to memory issues—what do we consider *issues*? So, when we come across studies that use terms that could be defined in various ways, we need to seek the study's definition. Do not rely on dictionaries; they are not significant in the context of research unless the study explicitly states that it is using a definition from the dictionary. This study, if it does use the dictionary, will not assume that one owns a dictionary; the definition will be, and should be, clearly stated.

Findings as they relate to life and longevity are complex. The stated article relating to order and achievement resulting in living longer is a complex finding in terms of interpretation, and the literature is split. For example, ambitious people can make more money, and ambitious people are less likely to live sedentary lives and are on-the-go. Impulsive people are more likely to engage in risky behaviors, and we know that accidental death is one of the most common causes of death. This could skew the data. When reviewing articles and studies, it is important to determine whether or not they had adequate sample sizes controlled for variables such as race, age, gender, personality features, socioeconomic status, and all other relevant variables. Not all studies will control for these variables, as it can be difficult in certain studies, but these are still important considerations in terms of drawing conclusions.

On the other hand, ambition in an incessantly changing landscape can have its downsides. Cortisol secretion, the stress hormone, negatively impacts health outcomes and can actually deplete certain brain networks of their reserves, no different than chronic stress or PTSD. Cardiovascular health is at risk, which is directly related to cerebrovascular risk because the heart supplies blood to the brain. Many variables are at play. Conscientiousness is known to improve health through a variety of means associated with this characteristic, along with vocational and educational success. While these traits are not protective factors in terms of depression or suicide alone, there are subcomponents that may serve as protective, such as diet, accomplishments, financial stability, sense of self, and other variables. However, when we are discussing research, we are referring to statistical significance rather than clinical significance. That which is the former may not guarantee clinical significance, and the reverse is also true.

Regret is the last term that seems appropriate in the context of the preceding chapter, which is another term that is defined differently by others. Many people claim that it is wrong to regret. Because some view regret negatively, regret seems as if one is ruminating about the past and not letting go and moving forward with life. Others, however, can accept that they regret certain acts and would take them back if they could, but they can't, so they accept that unassailable reality. They do not need to comfort themselves beyond knowing that this is the world in which they live. They regret some of it, they may regret more, but they try to keep that to a minimum moving forward. There is no right or wrong way to view this situation as long as one finds contentment. If one experiences significantly greater pain through regret, one may be better served by reframing it or changing how *regret* is viewed.

Resistance

I assess the power of a will by how much resistance, pain, torture, it endures and knows how to turn to its advantage

Friedrich Nietzsche

To me, the Nietzsche quote correlates "will" with "resistance." Throughout my long months of trouble, how much I could resist daily life or, to put it more accurately, the pain and hardship of daily life, was directly related to how much willpower I could muster each day. I am sure that question applies to anyone who is going through some level of hardship. And as much as I wish I could pretend I had some magic formula, I didn't and don't. In my case, each day was different, and it was different because the evils and demons with which I was fighting each day differed, and the degree of *their* persistence to keep me down varied from one day to another.

My day usually started with the mandatory two cups of coffee that I have to have in the morning. I would then spend a bit of time going through Internet sites of news organizations such as the *Washington Post*, *New York Times*, BBC, and Fox

News (to get the different sides). I would then sign into the Facebook, both to see what the people I know were up to and to see what news items people had posted as suggested reading. In the months preceding and following the US presidential elections, there were obviously massive numbers of suggestions. I did not read an overwhelming majority of them. First, I did not want to become as partisan and heated as some of the people I know had become. Second, I took care not to spend too much time away from the main task: looking for a job!

I had made this arbitrary rule for myself that I would apply to ten new jobs every day. Some days, it was easy to find that many new jobs. I had a fair number of websites that I visited, if not every day then every other day. I also had created job alerts on a number of sites that would send me suggestions for new jobs. Sometimes, it was fairly straightforward. You would attach your CV and cover letter, click the Send button and, boom, your application was off to the esteemed attention of someone who probably received over one hundred other such applications. But increasingly, companies and organizations want you to apply through their website and manually enter all your previous jobs, titles, duties, start dates, end dates, references, not to mention all the Equal Employment Opportunity questions for jobs in the

United States. Are you male? Yes! Are you Hispanic? No. Do you have disabilities? I often wanted to just be a smartass and say something like, "If you include mental incapacitation, yes!" But of course, they were only looking for a yes or no, and I am sure the dry sense of humor would not have carried over well in the first place. You fill out a few of those applications every day, and it becomes pretty tiresome after a while. Nevertheless, that is what I did every day, day after day, month after month.

But some days it simply was not easy to find new jobs. After all, there really are not *that* many jobs available in a given field, and when you apply for on average ten jobs a day, eventually the wells dry up. After a while, the task of finding suitable jobs becomes a mental and physical challenge in itself. That was not necessarily a bad thing. After all, I would like to believe that I thrive on challenge. In some weird and perhaps psychologically sick way, the fewer jobs there were, the more upbeat and motivated I became to find them! So, how much willpower I had at times depended on how much hassle I had to put up with to find ten new jobs. Most days, I could apply to that many jobs—and often even more—by 4 or 5 p.m., but sometimes it took longer and I would still be at my computer at seven, eight, or nine in the evening. Needless to say, by then I was pretty exhausted, both physically and mentally, especially when you end up doing it seven days a week for eleven *very* long months.

The willpower and ability to muster resistance power, however, often times is also directly related to one's psychological state. Whether I was in a good or bad state of mind was as much the question of my mood as whether I was turned down by a job I had really wanted, or whether the wait to hear back about a job was dragging me down, or whether someone had advertised for a job for which I had built up hope, only to hear that the jobs was canceled. Or whether it was none or all of the above. When it came to state of the mind, there was no telling why I became depressed or demotivated any given day. It just happened. And when it did, the willpower to resist just shrank or even went out the door.

Given all that was going on in my life, one thing I tried to continue doing steadfastly was exercising. I would not label myself a health nut or sports addict, but over the years I have become healthier and paid more attention to exercising. At some point in my life—perhaps as long as fifteen or twenty years ago—I was a regular tennis player. I was never particularly good at it, but I enjoyed the game nevertheless. I have not played in years, first because I hurt my knees and then because I was living in places where playing tennis was not all that conducive. Iraq, Afghanistan, Liberia, South Sudan, Yemen, etc., did not exactly cater to such outdoor sports. Running, whether on treadmill or in the street, has become more of a thing for me in the past decade or so, and I tried to pursue it as often as I could that year. One of the advantages of living in the South of France is that the area is perfect for many types of physical activities, including jogging and running. I have used the opportunity quite a lot. But I also had bought the treadmill so I could exercise at home if the weather was not agreeable outside, or if I was just too busy, or if I wanted to be nice to my knees.

Exercising did indeed change my mood—once I brought myself to doing it, when I was in the mood for it, or when I could force myself to change my mood by doing it. It was my way of increasing my own resistance level. I had placed the treadmill in one of my extra bedrooms on the first floor overlooking nothing but beautiful open space and hills surrounding the area. I must admit, just running on the machine, listening to some good music on my first-generation iPod, and gazing at the scenic scenery from the balcony gave me both motivation and a sense of temporary escape from the miseries of unemployment and everything else that came with it.

There was, however, another variable in my resistance level factor: my health. The second week of February, just about a month after I had left my previous job in The Hague, I was having a friend and her family at my house. They were leaving that morning. I tried to get out of the bed in the morning, rolled from one side to another, and with that slight move, I felt my head spinning like someone who was totally drunk and could not control his body. I felt it was strange and obviously did not like the feeling but thought it was something temporary. We had had wine with dinner the previous night. In fact, I remember we had started having a couple of glasses late in the afternoon after we returned home from a daytrip, but all together, I don't think I had more than four or five glasses over a period of five or six hours. I definitely was not drunk. When my friends left that morning, and I leaned against the heat radiator in the living room, facing the wall. In less than five seconds, I was losing my balance and was on the verge of crashing. I managed to quickly turn around and lean against the wall, letting my back provide the support that my brain was not offering. Then, I just stood there for seemingly a very long time. I could not move and felt so weak that I did not dare risk it. I lowered my back against the wall and the radiator slowly and managed to sit on the ground, took some deep breaths, and then moved on the floor while sitting and somehow, still sitting, climbed the stairs that led to the bedrooms. I made it back to my bed, felt my head spin fast again, and fell sleep.

To my own astonishment and anguish, I stayed in bed for the next three days. Every time I turned and tossed, my head would spin again, and I either could not or was scared of getting out of the bed, short of a few times that I had to get out, eat, or go to the bathroom. It was just short of a week that I felt stable enough to get up without having to go back to bed, but only to drive a relatively short distance to stock up on food and come back home. I got an appointment with a local doctor, who prescribed some pills, but after a week I was still the same.

What ensued were many months of back-and-forth trips from my house to Paris, a train journey of five and a half hours, to see specialists at the American Hospital in Paris. There were tests after tests, and audiograms after audiograms. At some point, the doctors were so concerned with the longevity of the vertigo they had diagnosed me with that they ordered an MRI to rule out a brain tumor. "Vertigo lasts a month or so," said one doctor at the time. "This could be something more serious." It was not. But the MRI did point to the degeneration of bones in the inner walls of my left ear. Next came more, and more, and more pills, none of which really made any inroads. As a last resort, they told me I must have a series of injections into my left ear, each within a couple of weeks, which meant going back and forth between my house and Paris. I have a few friends in Paris, but none had housing arrangements that could easily accommodate repeat guests. My bills were running up.

By the time I finally kicked the vertigo, it was around late September. However, the vertigo was substituted with tinnitus, that very annoying and continuous ringing in the ear. For the same reasons that my vertigo lasted longer than it should have, perhaps because of the other pressures that lowered my natural immune system, the tinnitus was not going away either. In fact, it has stayed with me, and it seems I have to deal with it for the rest of my life, although its intensity is not as bad, and most of the time my body has learned to ignore it.

Depending on how you would like to look at the situation, the combination of different types of pressure I was under was making me both more miserable and more resistant. At the end of the day, resistance became about one thing and one thing only: Do you have the hope that something better will—not might, but will—happen in the timeframe that is acceptable and feasible? If the answer is yes, then you wake up in the morning, you push on the resistance peddle, and hope for another day!

One of the most important ways of increasing resistance to the pressures of unemployment—something I tried to do occasionally but did not do on a consistent basis—was to create and maintain a decent work-life balance. Statistics show that, in the United States at least, the longer you are out of job, the longer it takes you to find a new job. That's just a general statement. Add to that the particulars of the case for any given individual—age, education, how specialized of a job you are looking for, how junior or senior of a job you are after, etc.—and those factors might make the process even lengthier. But keeping that work-life balance is easier said than done. We all have bills to pay. If you are supporting a family or someone else, you feel the pressure to meet your obligations. If you are single like me and have no backup financial support, you wonder how to deal with your obligations. But psychologists would tell you that doubling the number of hours that you sit behind a computer pushing out tailored CVs does not amount to a doubling of the number of good jobs you apply to, or good cover letters you write, because after a certain point our brains do not function as well. And the physical and psychological negative impacts carry on to the next day, and the effect compounds from one day to the next. Experts, as well as my chiropractor, say you should force yourself to quit working at your computer every two to three hours, take a twenty- to thirty-minute break, and stop working after between seven and ten hours. Just close the computer and call it a day!

The second thing that psychologists emphasize is to maintain a social circle—again, something I did not do. One of the easiest things to do when you are unemployed is to dig into your own shell and disappear. Between the pressures of finding a new job and the stigma attached to being unemployed—the shame of being unemployed, or the shame of having to explain why you are still unemployed after a long time—it is easy to not want to be in the presence of others, but part of the burden here falls on other people, people close to you. They are the ones who should also monitor the behavior of people who are in some kind of a trouble, make sure they don't disappear from the radar. If that circle is maintained, it strengthens the will to resist.

Another factor relevant in resistance is something I have mentioned before: choosing some short-term goals. Resistance is a day-to-day thing. There is no way of telling when you wake up in the morning whether it will be a good day or a bad day—or if a bad day, how much of a bad day; or if a good day, how long it will last. When you are in a prolonged struggle to find a new job, when you are worried about being in financial trouble and the psychological pressure is already building up, it would be rather helpful to bring in some positive energy to your-otherwise-miserable situation. While I had very few short-term goals—and therefore few "wins"—during the ordeal of 2016, I can attest from experiences during other periods in my life that it really does make a difference in one's mood and morale to feel good about having achieved something. We must also remember that psychological power is just like physical strength. You build it over time, bit by bit. So, having short-term goals and achieving short-term wins actually helps building internal resistance power, which in turn makes it easier to keep going and solve the big problem.

If only I had learned those lessons, or actually abided by them, myself when I was in real trouble!

Resistance

(By Jack Lennon)

Nietzsche's quote from the previous chapter includes the term *will*, which is a complicated one touched upon in previous chapters. It also requires an operational definition to fully understand what Nietzsche intended to say. We can only speculate as to his intentions based on what we know about his philosophies. One could speak ad nauseum about this term. It is possible that he was referring to resiliency. Will and willpower, at least from a scientific perspective, imply that one could change life if only he or she *chose* to do so. It is not uncommon to hear people claim that others with these health concerns lack willpower, which is not scientifically supported. This is arguably a major concern related to mental health. The stigma by which it is surrounded often makes people believe that they should be able to pull themselves out of a deep depression—they lack willpower if they cannot do so on their own. One can easily see how this view of oneself, and the views of others, could serve to worsen depression in those who do not accept the science of its occurrence.

In a previous chapter, we discussed behavioral activation—the forcing of ourselves to get up and do things that we may not be interested in doing but will still prove advantageous. This includes submitting job applications when we are feeling unmotivated. This chapter describes strong goal setting, including quantitative measures. A certain number of applications were expected to be submitted on a daily basis. This may need to be altered as the number of job openings changes, but this is an excellent example of keeping oneself on track with an ultimate goal in spite of the psychical pain being experienced. Goals can also be smaller or less taxing than those noted—this is a matter of trial-and-error. If one attempts a certain number of applications, or a number of anything, and it becomes too much to handle, it is both appropriate and clinically indicated to reduce that number. The ultimate goal is to make these small steps attainable so that the brain can recognize accomplishment each and every day. We do not want an individual to be disappointed with himself or herself because they could not achieve a certain goal. We want the goal to be met without worsening symptoms. One should test the self but know the limits.

Exercise, including walking, does alter mood on a molecular level, even if it is less noticeable on some days. The willingness to get up and exercise, or even take a walk, is another form of behavioral activation. The role of exercise as a life change during states of depression, sadness, anxiety, or other negative states cannot be understated. This is not to say that one must engage in exercise, which would depend on one's health status, but it is a worthwhile endeavor. When an individual becomes bedridden, unable to get out of bed for days at a time, this is the point at which one should seek assistance. This is a level of depression that may not warrant a diagnosis but does warrant a professional opinion. Again, and an important note, not everything out of the ordinary requires a diagnosis. One would not arbitrarily diagnose cancer or Alzheimer's disease without sufficient data, and depression should not be arbitrarily diagnosed without sufficient symptoms. But one can provide a substantial disservice to the self by not seeking assistance when life seems to be coming to a halt for more than a day or two in spite of one's desire to get out of bed.

Maintaining a social circle can be helpful during both the good and bad times. This is not always an easy task depending on the circle one has maintained over his or her life. While people experiencing depression can benefit greatly from having people for support, significant depression can counterproductively push people away. It is wise to maintain some form of social interaction when feeling down, however defined, but one should not overwhelm himself or herself with social interaction that becomes stressful. A small circle of people in whom one can trust is likely ideal for most people. If this is not the case for some people, requiring them to build a network, consider those people from the past who may be interested in starting fresh. If one wishes to remain separated from the past, finding new people might be the best option. Social media is not a replacement for in-person interactions and can easily become a problem, but it is not abnormal in this era to meet people through these mediums.

A last note regarding the ups and downs; it is important to reflect on how one views symptoms and whether or not they are skewed in the negative direction. For example, the previous chapter notes that when it's a bad day, we ask *how bad*. When it's a good day, we ask *how long it'll last,* rather than *how good*. We should attend to these thoughts and attempt to recognize how both low mood and clinical depression make people think, while actively working toward changing these thoughts to better reflect positivity. If one believes that good days are only a sign of impending problems, human beings have a tendency of making this true; this is not metaphysical, but instead an example of how thoughts alter our behaviors and, thus, our emotions. Our behaviors act in accordance with our thoughts, and vice versa, such that thinking more positively can prove advantageous in small ways that should eventually become second nature to us over time.

Shame

A painful feeling of humiliation or distress caused by the consciousness of wrong or foolish behavior; a regrettable or unfortunate situation or action

Merriam-Webster Dictionary

A painful feeling of having lost the respect of others because of the improper behavior, incompetence, etc., of oneself or another

Webster's New World Dictionary

More than dealing with the pain and physical near suffocation when bouts of sobbing came, the thing that was most difficult during my period of anguish was the pain of shame. I look at the question of shame in a similar manner as I look at hope: short term and long term. As a first-generation immigrant to the US, I take the idea of "making it" in my new homeland very seriously. It does not matter if I live in the States or overseas. It is the spirit of the cultural value that matters. I take a rather more rigid approach to this issue than many other immigrants I have met. To me, if you are adopting America as your new home, you'd better have a purpose in mind. You'd say, "Well, I want to have a better life." I'd say, "Okay, but that is not detailed enough. Who do you want to become and how do you plan to get there?" Almost like, "Show me the business plan."

I remember back in the 70s when I was a kid, my favorite TV show was an American miniseries, which in the States ran on ABC, titled *Rich Man, Poor Man.* The series were mainly about the ambitions of a young Rudy Jordache, played by Peter Strauss, who wanted to get elected to the US senate seat of his father after he passed away. To just about everyone in my family, I was a Rudy Jordache, a young and ambitious kid who would "go places." I even had a suede briefcase not much unlike what Jordache carried on TV. Of course, back then, no one was thinking of me going to America, much less becoming a US Senator. Except me. I don't remember if I thought or wanted to become a lawmaker, but I certainly saw myself in America and even considered studying law for many years.

So, I certainly won't deny that, sitting unemployed for an entire year in 2016, I grappled with disappointment bordering on shame at having squandered my decades struggling but not reaching any grandeur in either journalism, academia, or the UN. I questioned many things: my choices of professions; my own track record in each; and what I could have, should have done better or more so I could have become something or someone. As I said before, I am my own harshest critic, and that year I piled on myself much more than my physical, psychological, or financial strengths and means could handle.

There was also the short-term shame. I talked before a bit about "Are you good enough?" Very closely related to that is the sorrow that week in and week out, month in and month out, I was unable to find a job. I only had two or three interviews between January and October, having sent out close to two thousand CVs. There were two or three jobs in the States that either they did not follow up on or I did not pursue because both sides realized the salary was going to be rather tight for what I needed. Other than those, It was simply rejection letters (mostly from private sector companies in the States and internationally that probably did not find me suitable because I have never worked for a commercial or a for-profit company since I left my technical writing jobs with IT companies in 2003).

I am not sure which one was more pressuring: not receiving answers for all the good jobs I applied for and thus kept waiting and waiting and waiting, or being turned down for the extremely few jobs I was interviewed for. I suppose the latter. These were the jobs I really, badly wanted. These were the jobs for which I spent days preparing, understanding what the organization does (which I mostly knew because they were UN jobs), imagining the questions they might ask (the UN has something called competency-based interviews in which they ask hypothetical questions based on competencies such as professionalism, teamwork, or respect for diversity) and then writing down proper answers and rehearsing them until I had memorized them all.

But UN agencies also have a horrible habit. They advertise for a position, most probably give you a written exam, followed by an oral interview. At the end of each interview, they normally ask if you have any questions, and I normally ask, "When do you realistically think you might make a decision?" The typical answer is two to four weeks, which on the surface of it is okay—except it rarely happens that way. You wait and wait and wait. Sometimes months. Literally. Months, and no answer, and if you email and ask, "So, what's happening?", you get a generic and annoying human resources email saying something to the tune of "We cannot tell you anything. Just wait." To think that all these organizations bother to announce job vacancies, excite hundreds, sometimes thousands, of candidates to send in tailored cover letters and CVs, then go through at least two rounds of exams and interviews, and then sit on them for months and months is totally demoralizing.

What does it say about them that they cannot get their act together to finalize a simple hiring? If these organizations are so disorganized that they cannot manage a simple hiring process in a timeframe that they have committed themselves to, why should they expect applicants to be eager to work for them? But of course we do, because we are the beggars. We are the ones in need. We are the ones waking up in the middle of the night wondering when our savings will totally run out, and then wondering if you really will have to commit suicide because there is no other option left before you because there is no other way to pay the bills. Do the people on the other side think about those issue? Of course not.

All those issues and arguments aside, to be so utterly unable to find a decent job that pays what you can be happy with, the kind of job that you can be pleased with yourself doing day after day, and to fail to find such a job for many, many months is shameful. I am not passing judgment on other people, but I was ashamed of myself. Why is it that someone like me who has worked all his life, worked hard, was in that position? Remember what I said about "Am I paying for some past sins?" Even if that is the case, it is awesomely cruel that I had to be diminished to such a low point that I could not find a job and thus feel ashamed of myself.

I know a lot of people will say, "Oh, he's just saying this nonsense because he was depressed." But not so. First of all, I am writing these lines after I have passed the unemployed stage. Second, when I say I was ashamed, I am passing a professional judgement on myself. Nothing else. How is it—why is it—that someone who has managed to be gainfully—albeit at times unhappily—employed all his life, is all of a sudden found by thousands of employers across the globe unqualified? I have a colleague at one of the UN agencies in Geneva. I remember like it was yesterday when I called him after several months and the first thing out of his mouth was "You're calling *again* for a job?" Actually, that time I was not. I was calling just to say hello. I had called precisely because I was conscious of the fact that I indeed had sought his help many times—and he always felt too ethical to pull strings on my behalf. This time, I really had called to maintain the relationship and friendship, and I am absolutely positive he did not mean it in any negative way, but his words were like freezing-cold water on my soul. I don't think I will ever forget that call.

In the course of all those months in 2016, I also found that shame is more powerful, and more damaging, than pain. Some might find this odd, but it is true—at least it was for me. I have learned to tolerate pain for a few hours and it eventually will go away. I can cry my heart out, suffer the chest pain, the thought that I might physically not be able to inhale the next breath, but it will go away. Sometimes—not often at all—a couple of glasses of wine or maybe a whiskey also helped. But it went away, eventually, at least until the next time. Shame lingers. It lingers for days at a time, weeks at a time. And when weeks lead to months, it does not just increase proportionally. It compounds exponentially. And even when it leaves—if it leaves—it leaves a residue. When shame returns the next time, the lingering residue makes it even more powerful.

One of the reasons 2016 became more difficult as months went by was that the shame of unemployment was also changing my social character. When I was a kid and then in my younger years, I was more of an extrovert. I was never bubbly, but I actually liked being in large social gatherings. You could throw me in any large party, and I would be just fine. As I got older, I became less extroverted in some ways but more appreciative of smaller gatherings and establishing deeper bonds. Partly because of having worked in multiple countries in the past decades and therefore having made a lot of friendships, plus getting older—which I am told makes us naturally more conservative—I have had increased cravings for continuous friendships with only about a dozen people. They are the people who have been in my life for many years, whose friendship and love I cherish, and whose support I have needed and will undoubtedly continue to need. That is not to say I am not an extrovert anymore. I am, but in my professional life. When it comes to my personal life, I have become more inward-looking (and seeking).

Between the geography of where I was living in 2016—the South of France—and the shame of not having been able to find a new job, I found myself withdrawing from the world during those hard months, and more so as months went by. I withdrew from the world, from my circle of friends and acquaintances, bit by bit but ever so surely. Whereas I used to be good at sending emails, sending flowers for friends' birthdays, just being in touch, I was doing those things less and less that year. Even to the degree that I was keeping in touch, I could see that the tone of my emails had changed. Emails were shorter, the tone colder, sentences not nearly as warm. There are people I had always made a point of keeping in touch with, even if it was once every two or three months. I did not do that for probably six or seven months in 2016.

Of course, there is an argument to be had on why people don't keep in touch with you, don't keep an eye on you, don't provide more support, knowing you are in trouble. That is not a minor issue at all. The majority of family members and relatives concede *after* someone has committed suicide that they saw some level of withdrawal on the person's part but did not follow up. They just attributed it to "they were busy with their life and we were busy with ours. We did not see anything special in that." That is particularly true of youth and teenagers, where there is a natural gap between parents and kids at that age anyway. It is a sad fact of life that our lives have become more crowded, that we are busier than we used to be, but is that really a good excuse to give up on the people around us, people we say we care about, people we say we love? I don't think so.

I realize what follows is totally easier said than done, because I went through it myself, and I can attest that I did almost none of what I am about to say now. Having said that, there are a few things that might make the circumstances easier if we keep them in mind. They have to do with why we lose our job and why we cannot find a new one. Why is that important? Because while hindsight is 20/20, what I have to say might help some readers. I know I referenced some of this before, but it is really worth keeping in mind in these hard times for so many people around the world. There are many reasons why people lose their job, and knowing some of the background might ease the psychological pressure.

One of the hardest things for me to deal with during my ordeal, which prompted the chapter before on "Are You Any Good", was why I was ineffective in finding a new job. All the reasons I looked at were what I could call internal reasons, reasons that were specific to me: that my age was working against me; that my CV was not attractive for private commercial companies, even those with lots of international operations; and that I was a white male, American, and many international organizations were looking for more diversity and younger people. In the UN—though they would not admit it—there is actually an unwritten quota system. If there are already many Americans in a given office or the organization as a whole, they would prefer to take a less-qualified person from a country less represented. All of those are facts. But another side of the issue is how employment patterns have changed over time, and regardless of how qualified one might be, there may be times when one just has to look at career aspirations differently.

If you look at it from that perspective, hard as it might be to feel otherwise, one could rationalize that having become unemployed, or continuing to be unemployed, is to some degree because of factors outside our control, and therefore one should not feel as ashamed as she or he does. Again, I know it is easier said than done! I also know it only applies in some cases and to some people. I am not trying to generalize. It certainly did not apply to me when I lost my job in January 2016, but it did apply to why I did not get some of the jobs to which I had applied later that year.

In my case, to be fair, I was conscious of those factors, just as I was ashamed of myself. Being conscious of those factors helped somewhat, but it did not solve the problem. Everyone's case is different, and everyone must decide what is right for them. For me, I tried to adjust my employment requirements and aspirations as much as I could. As much as I wished I could continue to work with the United Nations, I diversified my search. I explored other areas. One of the fields that has grown a lot over the years is the work-from-home field. I figured I would be more than happy to stay home and take in writing and editing jobs, or do consulting work mostly from home but with occasional trips to wherever the employer wanted me to go. Although none of those ideas worked out for different reasons, I encourage readers to look into this field. It is growing by leaps and bounds every day, in part because employers find it cheaper to outsource than pay full-scale salaries, health benefits, vacation time, etc. Ironically, one of the reasons people like me cannot find high-salary professional jobs is because many employers, even large international organizations like the United Nations, are also taking the cheaper route!

There is a lot of literature out there about how and whether the Internet and other technological advances have cost people their solid, long-term, and blue-collar jobs. Whether artificial intelligence has or will replace human beings and cause more unemployment remains to be seen. The economy certainly has a lot to do with it, so does whether you are a man or a woman. I am not an economist, and I don't want to turn this chapter into discussing all factors affecting employment or unemployment, not to mention that most of the scientific and scholarly work is done in the United States and a few other Western countries, so I doubt anyone can talk definitively about the issue from a worldwide perspective.

The fact that world economic, social, and political changes have rattled employment patterns are undeniable, much more so since the outbreak of the coronavirus. The Organization for Economic Development in Europe, which actually looks far beyond Europe, had this to say in a report titled *"The Future of Work, OECD Employment Outlook 2019"*:

"We estimate that 14% of existing jobs could disappear as a result of automation in the next 15-20 years, and another 32% are likely to change radically as individual tasks are automated. Many people and communities have been left behind by globalization, and a digital divide persists in access to new technologies — resulting in inequalities along age, gender, and socio-economic lines . . . In some countries, for example, non-standard workers are 40-50% less likely than standard employees to receive any form of income support when they are out-of-work . . . The growth of inequalities of income and opportunities, distortions in cross-border competition, the perception of fiscal unfairness, the risk of climate change and the slowdown of the global economy, are all cause for concern . . . The key message of this OECD Employment Outlook is that the future of work is in our hands and will largely depend on the policy decisions countries make. It will be the nature of such policies, our ability to harness the potential of the unprecedented digital and technological change while coping with the challenges it poses, which will determine whether we succeed or fail."

And as for the reason I had become unemployed in the first place, to be brutally honest about it, I felt a hell of a lot more anger than shame. To some degree that was good, because I had recognized that I had not lost my job because I had made some gross error. Of course, we all make mistakes in our work or personal life, but I was pretty comfortable with myself that nothing I did at work was bad enough to deserve what I received. But I remained, and still am, rather angry with the people who put me in that situation: the two insane, disloyal, spineless, and incompetent people who showed no respect for other people as long as they could maintain their work turf and retain their cushy jobs and salary!

That brings me to the last topic before I end this chapter: the difference and relationship between shame and guilt. There was an online article by Dr. Robert D. Caldwell (http://www.psychsight.com/ar-shame.html) entitled *"Understanding How Shame Binds Us and How to Begin to Free Ourselves."* I learned that "Shame is the inner experience of being not wanted." It is feeling worthless, rejected, cast-out. "Guilt is believing that one has done something bad . . . There is nothing shameful about shame. You have every right to yours. You earned it by surviving in the midst of shaming people."

The article goes on to say, "**Replace shame with mature guilt.** Guilt has often received bad press, and well it should—if, and only if, you are talking about neurotic guilt—guilt that self-flagellates and changes nothing. If you are talking about mature guilt, then guilt is one of the great inventions of nature. For mature guilt lets you know what is unacceptable, and offers you opportunity to do something about it. Shame, on the other hand comes to you as a feeling so deep and so incapable of your getting a grasp on it that it seems there is nothing you can do."

I am not sure about the parts that say, "Shame is the inner experience of being not wanted," (except by myself at times) or that "You earned it by surviving in the midst of shaming people." I certainly never have meant to shame anybody else, but I agree with the broader conclusion that turning shame into guilt and then doing something about it is a good strategy. Although I am critical of myself for having changed course in life several times, I think *that* in itself was, perhaps psychologically, my way of turning guilt into action. Obviously, I have not achieved the end-results I wanted, but I think I have heeded the advice nevertheless!

Shame

(By Jack Lennon)

Guilt and shame are closely related but different; they can still be considered forms of pain. Guilt is remorse for wrongdoing, while shame is generally defined as a more severe and pernicious form of guilt, one that is characterized by negative feelings turned inward, whether it be perceived incompetence, immorality, or other inadequacies. It is unsurprising, based on what we know about negative thoughts and depression, that guilt and shame would both be major figures in the grand scheme of this book. Even if fault lies with other parties, rejection is likely to be turned inward to some degree. We may become extremely angry with the inadequacies or mishandlings of others, but we will not fall out of the equation. This is because we are also easy targets. We are the ones being rejected, often on several occasions, such that it does make some sense that we would look at ourselves to determine the flaws. The issues arise when our reflections change from trying to figure out how to improve job applications—or anything in life—to believing that we are innately ill-equipped based on the opinions of others.

We will experience frustration, hatred, anger, and sadness over the course of life. Even those who are capable of thinking positively in most situations are likely to have brief bouts of these states. The perfectionistic type will be displeased with this state of affairs—everything should be based on qualifications, desires, work ethic, and desire. The problem with this understandable viewpoint is that it is not a great fit with our reality. This realization could easily be painful, particularly if outcomes are not working in our favor. This does not mean that shame is different than pain—it is a form of pain. If one chooses to define pain in another way, that is perfectly acceptable, but generally unease and dissatisfaction could easily be considered pain in terms of one's mental health.

This chapter ultimately touches on the countless ways that one can view a situation. We can view a negative situation as it is—negative. We have the unique capacity to make negative situations seem even more negative than they are. We also possess the ability to denigrate the small, positive situations. It is not unusual to undermine the positive moments because we become so accustomed to finding negativity in outcomes. Over time, it can become increasingly difficult to feel pride for accomplishments, small or big. For those who are simply climbing the ladder and feel required to accomplish certain smaller goals to achieve an ultimate outcome, they may find little pleasure in those smaller accomplishments because they are mere stepping-stones. This train of thought may not cause harm, but it does set a precedent—*if I am not at my ultimate goal, my accomplishments do not matter.* The issue with this precedent is that, in this world, not everyone reaches that ultimate goal. Some discover a new, more rewarding, ultimate goal along the way, but the brain indiscriminately carries precedents over across situations. There may come a day when the ultimate goal also lacks a sense of pride because the goalposts have been moved to such a degree that one now wants more. This is not an ideal situation. Reflection is an amazing tool at our disposal, but it must be used appropriately and purposefully.

Leading a Double Life

I would very much like to tell you that the above title is going to lead you into a "007" chapter of my life and that I have some Roger Moore escapades I can recount, but that would be a lie. Although, throughout my journalistic career, I did collect enough material that helped me in writing my two fiction books! So, I am afraid "Leading a Double Life" is about something much more mundane.

I was not open about my suicide thoughts with that many people. I confided openly to a couple of friends and sort of insinuated to a couple of others about my thoughts and reasoning. I did not discuss it with more people for a few reasons.

First, I really am not and have not been looking for sympathy. Help maybe, although none of the people I confided in were in a position to pull some massive strings on my behalf, or that they would have done any less had I not confided in them. I suppose I also chose two of them because I knew they would understand that I am just trying to reach out without asking them to do anything, understand that I am not trying to self-grandiose, be melodramatic about it, or even ask them for money. They would have understood that I just needed to vent.

Second, and related to the first, is that I was not trying to unnecessarily worry people about something they could not—and I knew they could not—do anything about. No one around me was in a position to make someone else give me a job. So, why bother and worry people about something that is my problem, has nothing to do with them, and they cannot detrimentally change? I did not want to be selfish and just mess around with peoples' minds.

In all the literature I have read, and in the conversations I know of from just talking to people and observing life, people commit suicide because depression becomes too much to handle. For me, it was a purely financial matter. I was going to spend the money I had, or could even borrow, and then when it was over, it was going to be over. As I have said before, and this is just my personal opinion, and I am sure there are many people who would disagree, I am not a proponent of going to the degree of liquidating everything you have so you can live longer and restart your life again—maybe if I were thirty years old. I have led an adventurous life. I've covered wars, revolutions, popular uprisings, inhaled tear gas, managed not to get shot, and survived beatings by protestors and security agents. I have led a fuller life than most people can either dream of or would want to. If I find myself in such deep trouble that I see no way out, I will have no problem packing it in. No regrets.

What do I mean when I talk about leading a double life? There is no doubt that the experience I went through made me tired. I was demoralized. I felt a deep-seated sense of frustration and anger of having failed myself and my grand desires in life. But at the end of the day, I have never been the suicidal type, if there is such a thing. That dichotomy between the reality of the day and my own personality created such up-and-down months that on many occasions I felt like I was two different persons, often in the course of the same day. One minute you are fine, feeling upbeat, exercising, being creative in the cover letter you are writing in response to a job, appreciating that you are living in the South of France, and the next minute, boom, you are down, feeling tired, maybe crying your eyes out, and wishing this was your last moment on earth.

I am absolutely sure that I was not the only person living such a double life. I bet there are millions and millions of people who are going through the same emotions nowadays. They understand what I am saying. I learned a few lessons living those double-life moments. I realize these are all in retrospect and with 20/20 hindsight, but that is, after all, why Jack Lennon and I are writing this book: to hopefully provide insight that can help anyone who might be in the position I was in, or could use Jack's insight for any other problem for which these pages can provide help. These insights, however, are not a replacement for professional consultation or treatment, nor are they medical advice.

First, try to savor the good moments. You might not have too many of them. If possible, try to create more of them. If not, at least enjoy the ones you get. Do whatever pleases you. Listen to good music, stand in the middle of the living room and dance by yourself or with someone, tell your partner you love him/her and reminisce about good times, have a nice glass of wine, whatever pleases you. Having good moments in the middle of a crappy situation counts for something; even a few positive moments can boost your morale.

Second, when it gets really bad, stop whatever you are doing. I know fully well that it is much easier said than done, but you don't achieve anything when you are in that state of mind. Create diversions, just go to sleep, go for a walk, do anything but what you were just doing. It goes back to what I said in another part of this book: sitting at my computer for ten, twelve, or fourteen hours a day and just sending out CVs and cover letters did some harm to my own chances. I know it did. How? Because I went back and read some of those cover letters, and I found mistakes I know I would not have made in a different (read: better) state of mind.

That duality of the daily state of affairs must have affected my mind.

I think having that mix was inevitable. I am not sure how I could have avoided progressively feeling worse as months dragged on, but I think it was also good that I was able to include some positive thinking into it. Some of that was by necessity, I must admit. There were months after months that I was seriously concerned about the repercussions of the vertigo, the dizziness, and the at-times very menacing tinnitus, which, as I have said, I continue to suffer every day. Those concerns forced me to slow down a bit, to manage my anger and frustration, and the amount of time and energy I spent each day looking for a job. If that meant missing on the one job that could be saving me from having to take my own life, well, I guess I have become fatalistic enough to say, "So be it!", although I doubt that is ever the case. Forcing yourself to apply for one more job is more a matter of psychology than necessity.

Leading a Double

Life

(By Jack Lennon)

The incessant cycle of feeling a need to be physically and cognitively productive, only to feel better or worse based on that level of productivity, is the crux of emotional disorders. They often impact our abilities to engage in activities that would likely make us feel better. Essentially, they are self-perpetuating without an external force of some kind. This force could be in the form of changes in life circumstances, personal behaviors or thoughts, or positive life events. This also lends itself well to the well-supported cognitive-behavioral theory of how conditions arise and are treated. Thoughts (cognitions), behaviors, and emotions are interconnected, such that negative thoughts will worsen our feelings and alter our behaviors, thus perpetuating the endless cycle. We cannot always alter how we feel emotionally. We can, however, potentially alter how we behave (e.g., behavioral activation) and think (e.g., reframing situations, meditation techniques).

These could, in turn, change how we feel about a particular situation.

As we have discussed previously, the evidence suggests that there are unique neurobiological differences between those who are depressed, those who attempt suicide, and those who eventually die by suicide. There are far more attempts than there are deaths by suicide, and this is for a variety of reasons. Not everyone intends to die, not everyone engages in fatal means and are eventually saved via emergency medical procedures. On a more complex level, there appears to be differences on a molecular level that distinguish between these groups of people. It is not true that everyone must hit *rock bottom*; this term is intrinsically retrospective, in that it only exists in hindsight. One may say they are at rock bottom, but what does this actually mean? All it can logically mean is that the situation is worse than all other preceding situations; it is entirely possible that there are future moments that could be worse. It is a logical truth that one must reach a point at which it is believed that suicide is the appropriate behavior, but this need not follow a traumatic event or some highly negative experience. Suicide is a cause of death, but we are also on track to potentially consider suicidality as a path of its own, even separate to standard MDD or other disorders. Suicide is likely to involve mood disturbances, but this outcome is not seen in all who experience depressive disorders, even severe cases.

It is entirely possible that one may have never been the "suicidal type." One may or may not have met diagnostic criteria for Major Depressive Disorder or Persistent Depressive Disorder at some time, but that does not mean one was a suicidal type. It is entirely possible, in the evidence we have, that the suicidal type is special. One may not feel like that *type* but eventually might *become* the type based on the ongoing sequence of life events. There is some merit to this statement, irrespective of ups and downs, which is common in both depression and healthy life in general. However, this feeling should never outweigh our ability to engage in introspection, armed with the knowledge we have on depression and suicide, to understand when we have reached a point that warrants help from others, including professionals.

The reality is that life goes on. We continue to experience what life has to offer, and these experiences change us, for better or for worse. This is such a complex topic that we have not yet established ways to definitively determine who will and will not attempt suicide. We lack the ability to screen everyone who may need it due to healthcare disparities and a lack of targeted prevention methods. But as we continue to build upon our knowledge, and eventually translate our neuroscientific understanding of the brain to clinical practice, one must serve as his or her own advocate. Mental health is important, and the stigma is slowly diminishing in many cultures. Never let someone else determine what is right or wrong. The readers of these chapters are now prepared to engage in conversations with others and even mentor those who are experiencing these symptoms. It is perfectly acceptable to advocate for one's self by recognizing when problems are arising and seeking professional help. This does not imply that one will be forced to engage in treatment. One has the right to decide, and professionals will have the individual's best interests in mind. The literature supports the notion that a combination of therapy and medication is more effective than either one alone, specifically for those with severe symptoms. In less severe cases, therapy can often be the first course of action from a professional standpoint, and a discussion about medication can occur thereafter if therapy does not prove sufficient. Both routes take some time to prove effective, and it will still be expected that lifestyle changes occur during this time, if possible.

One should advocate for his or her own mental health with the same vigor with which one advocates for his or her professional life. The desired professional life cannot occur without mental health, no different than the need for physical health.

South of France: My Heavenly Hell!

On the surface of it, that chapter title is totally ludicrous, and I know it. After all, how could anyone say such a nasty—and untrue—thing about the south of France, or southern France? To be fair, the term "south of France" is somewhat misleading, because the southern part of France can be anywhere from the Atlantic Ocean on the western front to the world-renowned and glitzy Cannes, St. Tropez, and Monaco (which is not in France). If you drew a direct line between Biarritz—the farthest city on the lower west—to Menton—the farthest city in the east bordering Italy—the distance would be around 453 miles, or 730 kilometers.

But distance, of course, would be a terrible yardstick for measuring the enormity of southern France. The history, culture, arts, tourism, you name it, south of France has an exquisite and abundant treasure of them all. Much like many other countries in the world, there is also a wide cultural, linguistic, economic, social, and political gap between the south and the north, the east and the west. In the part that I live, there is a strong Catalan culture from the time much of this area was part of Spain. Many French friends from the north of the country have told me they have a hard time understanding people from this part of the south, especially the older generation, speaking their dialect of French, which has a different accent and many different words.

But not all of south of France is Cannes, Nice, or St. Tropez. Much of the beauty of southern France, or indeed France as a whole, is that it is full of small hamlets that have formed village after village. While some are closer to bigger cities and even bigger villages with easy access to main roads, shopping, and medical facilities, that is not the case for all of them. My house is in one such small village, with an official population of eighty and a pretty even mix of old French citizens and foreigners.

A bit of background: Circa 2007–08, I was teaching journalism and communications at a university in Dubai, the famous city in the United Arab Emirates known for its glitzy and posh lifestyle. Over the years, I had accumulated a bit of cash. The other thing you need to know to understand my actions a bit more is that I am one of those Americans who has become very international, perhaps a bit too much. I know a fair number of people like myself. We have lived outside the country for so long that for some odd reason we are more comfortable outside the United States. The America that I knew when I emigrated to in the 1980s is very different from the America we know today—or perhaps it was always the same and we just didn't notice. I could not but choke every time I watched the massive demonstrations I saw in the country in 2020 in the aftermath of an African American man choking to death at the hands of white police officers. Or the massive—and I really mean massive—queue of cars lined up in dozens of cities in the country so people could collect food baskets once coronavirus shut down much of America's economy. So many of us are so poor, living from paycheck to paycheck, that we ran out of money in less than a month once people lost their jobs. I hate to think this really was the America that millions of immigrants have idolized over decades and centuries.

So, while I have had my home right outside Washington, DC, for the past two decades, I had thought for years of having a second vacation home somewhere in Europe. I did not know where, as long as it was relatively close to the sea. That answers the often-asked question: "Are you a sea person or a mountain person?"

In my quest to find a new vacation home in Europe, or at least exploring the options, one summer break, I rented an apartment in Varna, on

Bulgaria's Black Sea. I chose the city because of its proximity—you guessed correctly—to the sea and because I thought housing there might fall within my budget, and also because I had some good Bulgarian friends at the time and thought it would be nice to be in a country where you actually know people with whom you can hang out. While I enjoyed my time and put thousands of miles on the rental car driving from the capital Sofia past Varna to the border with Romania, I decided against making Bulgaria my second home. It boiled down to two simple factors. First, the Varna area's per-square-foot price for constructed apartments and houses was way too high, not just for me at the time, but on par with more expensive parts of Europe. Second, because I do not have a European passport, it was literally next to impossible for me to get a loan to construct a house even if I paid cash for the land.

While I was in Bulgaria, a friend of mine and her husband who were my neighbors in the Washington, DC, area invited me to their house near the southern French city of Nice. They had bought a very old house in a nice, big village; the house needed a lot of work, and they had decided to do all the repairs themselves and live there for the rest of their lives. I accepted the invitation gladly. While I had been to Paris many times before, I had never been to the southern parts of the country. The vast, clean, green areas, beautiful scenery, and attraction after attraction raised my curiosity about the possibility of making France my second home. For the next year, every time I had time off from the university, I went to a different part of France to visit land plots I had already identified either through my own Internet search or through real estate agents with whom I had developed working relations. I simply flew to Paris, took a train to the nearest city, rented a car, and drove around. In the end, I settled on a midsize piece of land in my village about an hour's drive to the Mediterranean city of Perpignan, right across from the border with Spain.

I still remember my first impressions. The village was small, winding uphill for about ten minutes from a bigger village. I didn't see too many houses in the village. I did notice that there was no shopping facilities or a supermarket, not even a local bakery or butchery in the village, but at the time none of that bothered me. I bought the land because it had—and still has—a fantastic view. There is no construction in front of my house, and I have an absolutely open view into the lush green land—mostly in the summer, but also in the winter—and fabulous hills and mountain ranges. I was sold!

The fact is, I am still sold. I had to go through many hoops and challenges to get the house built, which I won't go into, but I still love my house and adore the location. To this day, sitting on my patio downstairs or on the balcony upstairs and looking into endless greenery or snow-capped mountains, clear blue skies or clouds moving as they block and unblock the sun changes my mood in an instant and gives me the tranquility I often need. The shortcomings, like having to drive ten minutes to buy anything, still do not bother me. Well, not much.

But the house was built to be the second home, somewhere I would go to stay on vacations, invite friends from all over the world so they could enjoy the beauty of south of France, and I would develop closer and better friendship with people I cared about. What it was not built for was what it became for the entirety of 2016: My permanent and primary place of residence where I *had* to live day in and day out, week after week, for the entire twelve months of the year. For that, I was not ready. For that, I had not signed up.

Still, I had to make it work. But how? At first, I tried to ignore the remoteness of the place. *Treat it like a normal office space,* I told myself. *Wake up in the morning, shave, shower, get changed, and work like it is normal work.* That should work, right? Not really. There were two problems. First, looking for a job day in and day out for months after months builds up the kind of internal pressure that is more powerful that sticks of dynamite. Pressure is inhibiting after a while. To compensate for that, you need some kind of "outing mechanism." When you are living in a small village, you have nowhere to go to release the pressure. Second, and because of the first, when the work part of the day is done, you are still sitting at home!

So, you realize that "after hours" or "evening hours" is basically "stay home" hours, just like the rest of the day. Therefore, you try to insert diversity in other ways. First, if there is nothing to do outside after hours, why not use the outdoors during daytime? Instead of staying home to work and look for a job during the day, you push some of that work to the afternoon and evening hours. You can then go out, walk, run, jog, or just drive around a bit during daytime. Certainly, in the spring and summer, there is plenty to do. The only problem with that was something I mentioned before in this book: the guilt factor. Psychologically, you cannot bear to go out and enjoy yourself even a bit, because, well, you should be home looking for a job, so you can earn money, pay the bills, and feel good that you are still a productive member of society.

Regardless of how you try to cut it, you realize after a while that living in a small village with nothing to do, having the pressure of having to find a job, and not wanting to go out and spend money on self-entertainment, dining, or what-have-you, the only way you can survive is by changing the routine on a regular basis, by breaking the monotony of life. Sometimes you wake up really early in the morning and go out running. Sometimes you sleep till ten so the day feels shorter. Sometimes you wake up normally, but instead of looking for a job, you simply become a couch potato and read for an hour and then work later into the evening. Other times you work till lunch and then hit the treadmill at the house and take a shower and continue working.

Of course, the house and its remoteness did provide the perfect excuse for me to hide in my own shell and withdraw from the world, simmer in my own juice, so to speak. It gave me the perfect excuse to hide my problems, my guilt, my shame, and my misery. It also gave me the excuse not to talk to people about planning for suicide.

Nevertheless, in the year that I was at the house, I pretty much tried any combination of events to make sure that I could insert and create as much diversity into my life as possible—not that it always worked. Often it did not, to the point where twice in 2016 I literally had to leave the whole area. In the summer and for the Christmas-New Year period, I was fortunate enough to have good and caring friends in Paris and Munich who allowed me to house-sit for them while they were on vacation. They will never know how much being able to live in a city meant to me—just living in a city environment, being able to walk the streets, walk or jog in parks, sit by street-cafés and have a drink, or just watch people go about their daily life. Those trips bought me back much of the mental sanity I had lost living in the village.

The point is—and I know this is a huge exaggeration and perhaps even a bad analogy—but living in a small village for someone who is pretty much a city boy is like forcing yourself to live in a prison-like condition. On the other hand, living in southern France when you are just on vacation and/or have money to go around and enjoy the vast and massively beautiful part of the world is a heavenly gift that not so many people can brag about. Now that my past troubles are behind me—and hopefully won't return—I consider myself extremely lucky, and I am grateful for the opportunity to live in this area. The small village part I will deal with in the coming years, hopefully.

South of France: My Heavenly Hell!

(By Jack Lennon)

Moving is considered one of the most stressful activities in which one can engage (McMahon et al., 2020). It is on the list with divorce, death of a loved one, and losing employment (Booth & Amato 1993). However, as is the case for everything in life, changing one's scenery may be for the best. It is likely that one will always find negative components of living in a particular area (the grass is always greener on the other side), but the ultimate goal is finding somewhere that provides the greatest good. Personal characteristics are important and should be considered, such as whether or not one prefers to be near people or away from them, near the water or city or away from them, near transportation and pleasurable activities or just far enough that one can walk to them. These are all considerations that are based on the individual.

Further, these thoughts and attributes may change over time. One may be interested in and prefer the city life and eventually become someone who prefers being away from the noise and lights.

Sometimes it takes a process of trial and error to determine what is best at a given point in time. If one feels that they are living in prison-like conditions, then that is the reality of the situation, even if one understands it to be hyperbolic. Sometimes it is not an exaggeration, depending on one's circumstances. One could certainly reframe this situation to the degree necessary to be content until changes can be made, but again, we must not invalidate our feelings simply because they seem exaggerated. Living with freedom is not the same as being in prison, but this does not change the feelings behind the statement. One must advocate for himself or herself; one must attempt to claim that which makes him or her happy. If several moves have not improved upon one's mood and he or she still feels trapped, then this is the point at which one must consider whether or not location is the primary concern.

Now that we are better informed and possess the skills necessary to recognize problems as they arise, and we understand that mental health is to be cherished and cared for, we can make informed decisions and learn as one proceeds down his or her chosen path. As deserving human beings, viable mentors, nonjudgmental friends, and informed citizens, we can venture down these paths with the necessary tools to care for ourselves and others when necessary.

References

Booth, A., & Amato, P. (1993). Divorce, residential change, and stress. *Journal of Divorce & Remarriage, 18*(1-2), 205-214. https://doi.org/10.1300/J087v18n01_10

McMahon, G., Creaven, A., & Gallagher, S. (2020). Stressful life events and adolescent well-being: The role of parent and peer relationships. *Stress & Health: Journal of the International Society for the Investigation of Stress*. Advance online publication. https://doi.org 10.1002/smi.2923

ABOUT THE AUTHORS

Peyman Pejman is an award-winning print and broadcast journalist, a communications officer for various United Nations agencies, and a university teacher of communications, media, and journalism.

He has more than two decades of experience with media organizations such as the *Washington Post*, The Associated Press, United Press International, Voice of America Radio, and Radio Free Europe/Radio Liberty. During his career, he covered many of the events that have marked the political scenery of the Middle East—and affecting other parts of the world—ranging from the Iranian Revolution and the 1982 Israeli invasion of Lebanon to the rise of Hizbullah, Hamas, or the Taliban.

He also has served in various communications capacities with UN agencies such as the Department of Peacekeeping, International Organization for Migration, UN Habitat, UN Food and Agriculture Organization, UN Office of Coordinator for Humanitarian Affairs, and United Nations Development Programme.

To Suicide and Back is his third book. He has previously published two fictions based on international current affairs topics titled ***The Age of Intolerance*** and ***The Misfit Radical.***

Jack C. Lennon is a researcher and doctoral candidate in Clinical Psychology and Neuropsychology. He engages in both clinical work with individuals with neuropsychiatric and neurologic conditions as well as multidisciplinary research that attempts to bridge the gaps in our understanding of suicide and neuropathology. His interests extend to the neuropsychology of suicide and using big data to optimize machine learning techniques for the prediction of future suicide attempts as well as disease trajectory. He has been published in various peer-reviewed medical journals and serves as a reviewer for several journals spanning the neurosciences and psychiatry. He is also heavily involved in leadership roles across several clinical disciplines and professional organizations and is a contracted writer for a medical publishing company.